Shulamith Lala Ashenberg Straussner
Christine Huff Fewell
Editors

Impact of Substance Abuse on Children and Families: Research and Practice Implications

Impact of Substance Abuse on Children and Families: Research and Practice Implications has been co-published simultaneously as *Journal of Social Work Practice in the Addictions,* Volume 6, Numbers 1/2 2006.

*Pre-publication
REVIEWS,
COMMENTARIES,
EVALUATIONS . . .*

"A DIVERSE REVIEW of the literature and current studies that speak to the legitimacy and urgency of the needs of families and children impacted by alcohol and/or drug abuse. . . . OFFERS THE READER AN IMPORTANT DISCOURSE FOR THOUGHT regarding research and practice. Particularly important is the implicit message that children and families are specific client populations that cannot and should not continue to be neglected."

Claudia Black, PhD, MSW
Author of It Will Never Happen To Me,
Specialist in families impacted by addiction

Impact of Substance Abuse on Children and Families: Research and Practice Implications

Impact of Substance Abuse on Children and Families: Research and Practice Implications has been co-published simultaneously as *Journal of Social Work Practice in the Addictions*, Volume 6, Numbers 1/2 2006.

Impact of Substance Abuse on Children and Families: Research and Practice Implications, edited by Schulamith Lala Ashenberg Straussner, DSW, CAS, and Christine Huff Fewell, PhD, CSW, CASAC (Vol. 6, No. 1/2, 2006). *Addresses the growing concern over children at risk of developing physical and mental health problems because of their parents' addictions to alcohol and other drugs (AOD).*

Substance Abusing Latinos: Current Research on Epidemiology, Prevention, and Treatment, edited by Mario R. De La Rosa, PhD, Lori K. Holleran, PhD, Shulamith Lala Ashenberg Straussner, DSW, CAS (Vol. 5, No. 1/2, 2005). *Examines the latest information, research, and recent advances in the prevention of substance abuse and HIV/AIDS in Latino populations.*

International Aspects of Social Work Practice in the Addictions, edited by Shulamith Lala Ashenberg Straussner, DSW, CAS, and Larry Harrison, MA, CQSW (Vol. 2, No. 3/4, 2002). *"Provides valuable insight into one of the most significant changes in social life during the last fifty years and indicates some of the likely direction for changes in the first half of the twenty-first century." (Tony Clamp, DipCouns, DipSW, MA, Lecturer in Applied Social Studies, University of Durham, United Kingdom)*

Neurobiology of Addictions: Implications for Clinical Practice, edited by Richard T. Spence, PhD, MSSW, Diana M. DiNitto, PhD, and Shulamith Lala Ashenberg Straussner, DSW, CAS (Vol. 1, No. 3, 2001). *Presents the neurobiological theories of addiction in a psychosocial context and connects the theoretical information with practical applications.*

Impact of Substance Abuse on Children and Families: Research and Practice Implications

Shulamith Lala Ashenberg Straussner
Christine Huff Fewell
Editors

Impact of Substance Abuse on Children and Families: Research and Practice Implications has been co-published simultaneously as *Journal of Social Work Practice in the Addictions,* Volume 6, Numbers 1/2 2006.

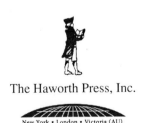

The Haworth Press, Inc.

New York • London • Victoria (AU)
www.HaworthPress.com

Published by

The Haworth Press®, 10 Alice Street, Binghamton, NY 13904-1580 USA

Impact of Substance Abuse on Children and Families: Research and Practice Implications has been co-published simultaneously as *Journal of Social Work Practice in the Addictions* Numbers 1/2 2006.

The development, preparation, and publication of this work has been undertaken with great care. However, the publisher, employees, editors, and agents of The Haworth Press and all imprints of The Haworth Press, Inc., including The Haworth Medical Press® and Pharmaceutical Products Press®, are not responsible for any errors contained herein or for consequences that may ensue from use of materials or information contained in this work. With regard to case studies, identities and circumstances of individuals discussed herein have been changed to protect confidentiality. Any resemblance to actual persons, living or dead, is entirely coincidental.

The Haworth Press is committed to the dissemination of ideas and information according to the highest standards of intellectual freedom and the free exchange of ideas. Statements made and opinions expressed in this publication do not necessarily reflect the views of the Publisher, Directors, management, or staff of The Haworth Press, Inc., or an endorsement by them.

Cover design by Lora Wiggins

Library of Congress Cataloging-in-Publication Data

Impact of substance abuse on children and families: research and practice implications /Shulamith Lala Ashenberg Straussner, Christine Huff Fewell, editors.
    p. cm.
    "Impact of substance abuse on children and families : research and practice implications, Volume 6, numbers 1/2 2006."
    Includes bibliographical references and index.
    ISBN-13: 978-0-7890-3343-7 (hard cover : alk. paper)
    ISBN-10: 0-7890-3343-7 (hard cover : alk. paper)
    ISBN-13: 978-0-7890-3344-4 (soft cover : alk. paper)
    ISBN-10: 0-7890-3344-5 (soft cover : alk. paper)
    1. Substance abuse–Social aspects 2. Substance abuse–Research. I. Straussner, Shulamith Lala Ashenberg. II. Fewell, Christine Huff. III. Journal of social work practice in the addictions.
HV4998.I54 2006
362.29′13–dc22
                                         2006002012

Indexing, Abstracting & Website/Internet Coverage

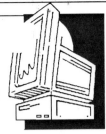

This section provides you with a list of major indexing & abstracting services and other tools for bibliographic access. That is to say, each service began covering this periodical during the year noted in the right column. Most Websites which are listed below have indicated that they will either post, disseminate, compile, archive, cite or alert their own Website users with research-based content from this work. (This list is as current as the copyright date of this publication.)

(continued)

Special Bibliographic Notes related to special journal issues (separates) and indexing/abstracting:

- indexing/abstracting services in this list will also cover material in any "separate" that is co-published simultaneously with Haworth's special thematic journal issue or DocuSerial. Indexing/abstracting usually covers material at the article/chapter level.
- monographic co-editions are intended for either non-subscribers or libraries which intend to purchase a second copy for their circulating collections.
- monographic co-editions are reported to all jobbers/wholesalers/approval plans. The source journal is listed as the "series" to assist the prevention of duplicate purchasing in the same manner utilized for books-in-series.
- to facilitate user/access services all indexing/abstracting services are encouraged to utilize the co-indexing entry note indicated at the bottom of the first page of each article/chapter/contribution.
- this is intended to assist a library user of any reference tool (whether print, electronic, online, or CD-ROM) to locate the monographic version if the library has purchased this version but not a subscription to the source journal.
- individual articles/chapters in any Haworth publication are also available through the Haworth Document Delivery Service (HDDS).

Impact of Substance Abuse on Children and Families: Research and Practice Implications

CONTENTS

ABOUT THE EDITORS

Shulamith Lala Ashenberg Straussner, DSW, CSW, CEAP, BCD, CAS, is Professor at New York University School of Social Work and Director of their Post Master's Certificate Program in the Clinical Approaches to Addictions. She was a Fulbright Senior Scholar to Israel in 2003; Distinguished Visiting Professor, Ben Gurion University, Israel, in January 2002; and Visiting Professor, Omsk State Pedagogical University in Siberia, Russia, Spring, 2000.

Dr. Straussner has numerous publications dealing with substance abuse. Among her thirteen books are: *Clinical Work with Substance Abusing Clients* (Guilford Press, 1994/2004); *International Aspects of Social Work Practice in the Addictions* (co-edited with L. Harrison, The Haworth Press, Inc., 2003); *Understanding Mass Violence: A Social Work Perspective* (co-edited with Norma Phillips, Allyn & Bacon, 2003); *The Handbook of Addiction Treatment for Women* (co-edited with Stephanie Brown, Jossey-Bass, 2002); *Ethnocultural Factors in Addictions Treatment* (Guilford Press, 2001); and *Gender and Addictions: Men and Women in Treatment* (co-edited with E. Zelvin, Jason Aronson Press, 1997). She is the founding editor of the *Journal of Social Work Practice in the Addictions* (The Haworth Press, Inc.).

Dr. Straussner is Regional Director, Project MAINSTREAM, a HRSA/CSAT/AMERSA sponsored national project to expend interdisciplinary AOD training within 17 different health and mental health professions. She has served on the National Center on Substance Abuse Treatment, panel on workforce issues and is a founding board member of the New York State Institute for Professional Development in Addictions. Dr. Straussner is the past chair of NASW Section on Alcohol, Tobacco, and Other Drugs. She received the Social Worker of the Year Award from the NASW ATOD Section in 2000 and Award for Individual Distinction in Addictions Education and Training from NY State IDPA in 2003.

Dr. Straussner serves as a consultant to various hospitals and other organizations and lectures on a variety of topics throughout the U.S. and abroad. She is trained in psychoanalytic psychotherapy, family, and group therapy and has a private clinical and supervisory practice in New York City.

Christine Huff Fewell, PhD, LCSW, CASAC, is Adjunct Assistant Professor, New York University School of Social Work and Associate Editor of the *Journal of Social Work Practice in the Addictions.* Her dissertation studied attachment and psychological distress in college-age children of alcoholics. Her professional activities and publications have centered on colleague assistance for social workers with alcohol and drug problems and working with substance-abusing families and adult children of alcoholics. Dr. Fewell is a graduate and member of the Institute for Psychoanalytic Training and Research (IPTAR) and the International Psychoanalytical Association and maintains a private practice doing psychotherapy and supervision in New York City and Westchester County.

Preface

Alcohol and drug dependence are pervasive international problems that severely affect the physical and mental health of the individuals who have them, their family members, and especially, the vulnerable children who are at risk of developing physical and mental health problems and substance abuse because of their parents' addictions. In contrast to the magnitude of the problem, little recent research and practice literature addresses these issues. To begin to address this gap this volume brings together current research and practice papers from authors in the United States, Ireland, Israel, and Australia.

In the United States, an estimated 21.6 million (9.1 percent) individuals were considered to have a substance use disorder in 2003. Nearly 15 million of these had alcohol dependence and nearly 4 million had drug dependence, while approximately 3 million had disorders related to both alcohol and drugs (Substance Abuse and Mental Health Services Administration [SAMHSA], 2004). Of all those in need of substance abuse treatment, only 3.3 million received it. Co-occurring mental illness and substance dependence presents an even more complicated situation, with approximately 21 percent of people with serious mental illness also reporting alcohol and drug use disorders (SAMHSA, 2004).

Parental alcohol and other drug abuse also have an enormous impact on children and adolescents in this country. Almost one-quarter of children in the U.S. (24 percent) lives in a household where a parent or other adult is a heavy or binge drinker (17 million) (The National Center on Addiction and Substance Abuse [CASA] at Columbia University, 2005).

[Haworth co-indexing entry note]: "Preface." Ashenberg Straussner, Shulamith Lala, and Christine Huff Fewell. Co-published simultaneously in *Journal of Social Work Practice in the Addictions* (The Haworth Press, Inc.) Vol. 6, No. 1/2, 2006, pp. xxi-xxviii; and: *Impact of Substance Abuse on Children and Families: Research and Practice Implications* (ed: Shulamith Lala Ashenberg Straussner, and Christine Huff Fewell) The Haworth Press, Inc., 2006, pp. xiii-xix. Single or multiple copies of this article are available for a fee from The Haworth Document Delivery Service [1-800-HAWORTH, 9:00 a.m. - 5:00 p.m. (EST). E-mail address: docdelivery@haworthpress. com].

xiii

More than one in 10 children lives in a family where illicit drugs are used (12.7 percent, 9.2 million) (Grant, 2000).

Living with a parent who is actively abusing alcohol or other drugs causes stress for all members of the family, including very young children. Parents are often unable to be consistently available, either because of their own use or their preoccupation with a partner's use (Zucker, Ellis, Bingham, & Fitzgerald, 1996). The cognitive developmental immaturity of children makes it impossible for them to accurately interpret the fact that the behavior of their parents is being influenced by the pharmacological action of mood-altering substances such as alcohol and other drugs (Markowitz, 2004).

Research has shown that many children are at high risk when they grow up with parental AOD problems. Children of alcoholics (COAs) are between four and nine times as likely to develop an alcohol use disorder as other children (Adger, 2000). They are also at risk for other mental health problems. Studies indicate that children of alcoholics tend to have two types psychiatric disorders: internalizing behavior problems such as depression or anxiety, or externalizing behavior problems such as attention deficit hyperactivity disorder, conduct disorder, and oppositional defiant disorder (Clark, Moss, Kirisci, Mezzich, Miles, & Ott, 1997; McConaughy & Achenbach, 1994). Externalizing behavior disorders are more commonly found in boys and internalizing behavior disorders in girls. Both have been found to increase the risk for substance abuse (CASA, 2003a).

Children of illicit drug abusers are more likely than other children to demonstrate immature, impulsive or irresponsible behavior, to have lower IQ scores, poorer school attendance, and to have behavioral problems, including depression and anxiety (Bauman & Dougherty, 1983). In addition, they manifest negative self-concepts, fearfulness, loneliness, difficulty concentrating and difficulty completing work (Fisher & Harrison, 2000). All of these put them at high risk for substance abuse (Bauman & Dougherty, 1983). The considerable shame and stigma associated with AOD problems make their identification difficult, and often requires skillful screening that takes into account the developmental level of the child or adolescent, as well as direct and indirect indicators. (Robinson & Rhoden, 1998).

Since its beginning, the social work profession has been in a position to interact with individuals, families, and children affected by alcohol and drug problems. As early as 1917, Mary Richmond, who made great contributions to the professionalism of social work in her groundbreaking book *Social Diagnosis* (Richmond, 1917), reframed the prevailing view of alcoholism as a moral weakness to one of a disease and created a diagnostic questionnaire that included assessment of family, medical, and psychiatric history, and current social, employment, and family situation (Straussner, 2001; Straussner & Senreich, 2002). Among other early social work contributions were those made by Gladys Price in her work with wives of alcoholic husbands (Straussner & Fewell, 1996) and Margaret Bailey with her monograph *Alcoholism and Family Casework* (1968). Margaret Cork, a social worker at the Addiction Research Foundation in Toronto, Canada first brought attention to the impact of parental alcohol problems on children in her book *The Forgotten Children* (1969).

Today, social workers encounter families with parental alcohol and other drug (AOD) problems in many settings. A national survey conducted by NASW (National Association of Social Workers, June 2, 2000) found that 40% of social workers were employed in mental health, 25% in child/family welfare, 12% in health, 5% in schools, 4% in aging, 1% in criminal justice, and 12% in other settings, including substance abuse. Thus, the majority of social workers are not employed in areas where AOD users and their children might be readily identified (Straussner & Senreich, 2002). It is likely that substance abusers and/or their children will seek care in medical and mental health settings where they are less likely to encounter professionals with alcohol and drug abuse expertise (Hall, Amodeo, Shaffer, & Vander Bilt, 2000). It is these social workers who are most in need of education about AOD problems and how to intervene most effectively with family members.

Yet, despite the research findings indicating serious consequences to many children growing up with parental substance abuse, there is a dearth of training available in social work schools. A recent review of courses at eleven major schools of social work was undertaken by Straussner to see if there were any courses dealing with children of alcohol and/or drug abusing parents. No course titles relating specifically to this population were found. To address this lack of training, the National Association of Children of Alcoholics (NACoA) began a Social Work Initiative in June 2005 which brought together social work educators, practitioners, researchers, prevention professionals, government representatives, and staff from the Council on Social Work Education. These meetings identified core competencies needed to work with children from alcohol and drug abusing homes and planned strategies for infusing knowledge, skills and attitudes into the social work curriculum and into continuing education for practicing social workers (for further information, see <www.nacoa.org>).

The papers included in this volume review the literature on children and families and point to areas needing further exploration and research.

Gruber and Taylor describe the rationale for using the family unit as an essential focus for examining the course and impact of substance abuse and review studies that describe the effects of substance abuse on the marital relationship and parenting practices of both male and female substance abusers. They highlight research on the emotional and behavioral problems experienced by children with alcohol and/or other drug abusing parents at different developmental periods, from prenatal exposure through adolescence. The important role that family members play in addressing (or not addressing) substance abuse and in providing support for recovery is emphasized. The paper concludes with recommendations for increasing the research focus on a family systems perspective and for including the family in treatment programming.

The disjuncture between research findings supporting the efficacy of marital therapy with alcohol abusing couples and the scarcity of its inclusion in treatment programs led Loughran to review the prevailing theoretical models on this topic in the literature of each decade from 1950s to the present. Reflecting the prevailing psychodynamic theoretical models of the time, the 1950s focused on the personalities of wives of alcoholics. The next two decades involved a move in the direction of family systems work. The 1980s reflected an interest in treatment outcomes and behavioral marital therapy. In the 1990s Project MATCH, which included no marital interventions, dominated the research agenda. In recent years, the interest in social networks and community reinforcement once again raises the possibility that the role of interpersonal relationships in maintaining substance abuse or supporting recovery might become of interest.

How does research inform our understanding of the impact of substance abusing parents on children? Peleg-Oren and Teichman's review focuses on 10 scientific studies done in the last two decades that investigated the impact of parental substance abuse on school-age children. These studies reported that a variety of emotional, cognitive, behavioral, and social problems were experienced by these children. Children of drug abusers were at higher risk than children of alcoholics for psychopathology and functional impairments. Children whose parents were also diagnosed with anti-social personality disorder were at special risk of negative psychosocial outcomes.

The increase in methamphetamine abuse during the last decade, particularly among women of childbearing age, has lead to reports of children being physically and emotionally neglected and exposed to serious environmental hazards, such as dirty needles and toxic materials. Brown and Hohman's qualitative study of 10 methamphetamine-abusing parents (including 3 fathers) provides one of the first efforts to investigate the impact of methamphetamine addiction on their parenting skills and their children. The identification of common detrimental parenting practices leads the authors to recommend comprehensive family recovery planning that include family and marital treatment, including parenting classes and on-site childcare.

Attachment theory and research is gaining increasing recognition as a valuable conceptual foundation for understanding and planning interventions with substance-abusing clients and their partners and children. Finzi-Dottan and colleagues have further added to this knowledge with their research on family characteristics and parental attachment styles on the children in a sample of Israeli drug using (DU) fathers who were participating in a rehabilitation program. The important effects of different combinations of attachment styles and their implications for clinical practice are discussed.

Residential treatment for drug abusing mothers and their young children is a treatment model that has developed in recent years in an effort to consider substance-abusing women's parenting needs while they are in treatment. However, the kind of social support provided and the way it is perceived by the mothers has only been explored in a very limited way. Wong's qualitative study examines the experiences of ten mothers residing in residential drug treatment facilities to investigate their perceptions of social support received from the treatment program. Important programmatic, policy, and research implications of the study's findings are discussed.

How can those children of alcohol and drug abusing parents most in need of intervention be identified at the time parents' access treatment? As part of a larger research project targeting a prevention and early intervention program for 4-13 year old children with substance dependent parents in Australia, Gruenert, Ratnam, and Tsantefski, evaluate the validity of a brief screening tool called the Strengths and Difficulties Questionnaire (SDQ) to assess its utility in identifying children most in need of help. They found that for the 48 children evaluated, significant and moderate correlations between SDQ scores and social workers' assessments of children's social, emotional and cognitive development and schooling. They conclude that the SDQ provided a quick and cost effective way to effectively and validly screen for children's problems at the time parents assessed drug treatment.

Leichtling and colleagues explore treatment outcomes for adolescent children of addicted parents in outpatient substance abuse treatment. While these adolescents enter treatment with greater problem severity, outcomes are similar to adolescents with no substance-abusing parents.

The impact of family and individual counseling on outcomes is also examined.

The school setting has been one of the primary sites for provision of services to children affected by parental AOD through programs such as Student Assistance Services on the junior and high school levels. The Special Topic of this issue is an interview of Ellen Morehouse by Lori Holleran, which describes the Westchester County (New York) Student Assistance Program founded by Morehouse in 1979. The program adapted the Employee Assistance Program model used to help employees in the workplace for use in secondary schools. Two additional models have been implemented, one for adolescents placed in residential childcare facilities (Residential Student Assistance Program or RASP) and an adaptation for use in alternative schools (Schools Utilizing Coordinated Community Efforts to Strengthen Students or Project SUCCESS). All three programs have been identified as national models by the National Institute of Alcohol Abuse and Alcoholism [NIAAA].

Finally, the Endpage by Zelvin compares and explores the themes and interventions emerging from Internet treatment of partners and adult children of alcoholics.

We hope that this special volume addressing the research and clinical implications of the impact of substance abuse on couples, families, and children will make an important contribution to the current limited social work literature on this important topic.

REFERENCES

Adger, H, (2000). Children in alcoholic families: Family dynamics and treatment issues. In S. Abbott (Ed.), *Children of alcoholics: Selected readings, Volume II,* (pp. 385-395). Rockville, MD: National Association of Children of Alcoholics.

Bailey, M. (1968). *Alcoholism and family casework: Theory and practice.* New York: Community Council of Greater New York.

Bauman, P.S., & Dougherty, F.E. (1983). Drug-addicted mothers' parenting and their children's development. *International Journal of the Addictions, 18*(3), 291-302.

Clark, D.B., Moss, H.B., Kirisci, L, Mezzich, A.C., Miles, R., & Ott, P. (1997). Psychopathology in preadolescent sons of fathers with substance use disorders. *Journal of the American Academy of Child and Adolescent Psychiatry, 36* (4), 495-502.

Cork, R. M. (1969). *The forgotten children.* Toronto: Paperjacks.

Fisher, G.L., & Harrison, T.C. (2000). *Substance abuse: Information for school counselors, social workers, therapists, and counselors* (2nd Ed.). Boston: Allyn & Bacon.

Grant, B. F. (2000). Estimates of U.S. children exposed to alcohol abuse and dependence in the family. *American Journal of Public Health, 90*(1), 112-115.

Hall, M.N., Amodeo, M., Shaffer, H.J., & Vander Bilt, J. (2000). Social workers employed in substance abuse treatment agencies: training needs assessment. *Social Work, 45* (2), 141-154.

McConaughy, S.H., & Achenbach, T.M. (1994). Co morbidity of empirically based syndromes in matched and general population and clinical samples. J*ournal of Child Psychology & Psychiatry, 35*(6), 1141-1157.

Markowitz, R. (2004). Dynamics and treatment issues with children of drug and alcohol abusers. In S. L. A. Straussner (Ed.), *Clinical Work with Substance-Abusing Clients.* 2nd ed. (pp. 125-145). New York: Guilford Press.

National Association of Social Workers (June 2, 2000). *NASW Demographic Status Report on Major Practice.* Unpublished report. Washington, DC: National Association of Social Workers.

O'Rourke, K. (1990). Recapturing hope: Elementary school support groups for children of alcoholics. *Elementary School Guidance and Counseling,25.* 107-115.

Richmond, M.E. (1917). *Social Diagnosis.* New York: Free Press.

Robinson, B., & Rhoden, J. L. (1998). *Working with children of alcoholics. Second edition.* Thousand Oaks: California: Sage Publications.

Straussner, S.L.A. (2001). The role of social workers in the treatment of addictions: A brief history. *Journal of Social Work Practice in the Addictions, 1*(1): 3-9.

Straussner, S.L.A., & Fewell, C. (1996). Social work perspectives on alcohol and drug abuse problems. In Kinney, J. (Ed.), *Clinical manual of substance abuse.* 2nd ed. (pp. 140-146). St. Louis, MO: Mosby

Straussner, S.L.A., & Senreich, E. (2002). Educating social workers to work with individuals affected by substance use disorders. *Substance Abuse, 23* (3), 319-340.

Substance Abuse and Mental Health Services Administration (2004). Overview of Findings from the 2003 National Survey on Drug Use and Health (Office of Applied Studies, NSDUH Series H-24, DHHS Publication Ni. SMA 04-3963). Rockville, MD. (Available at *http://oas.samhsa.gov.nhsda/2k3Overview.htm.* Retrieved 6/21/05).

The National Center on Addiction and Substance Abuse (CASA) at Columbia University. (2003a).The formative years: Pathways to substance abuse among girls and young women ages 8-22. New York: The National Center on Addiction and Substance Abuse (CASA) at Columbia University.

The National Center on Addiction and Substance Abuse (CASA) at Columbia University (2005). Family matters: Substance abuse and the American family. New York: The National Center on Addiction and Substance Abuse (CASA) at Columbia University.

Zucker, R.A., Ellis, D.A., Bingham, C.R., & Fitzgerald, H.E. (1996). The development of alcoholic subtypes: Risk variations among alcoholic families during the childhood years. *Alcohol, Health & Research World, 20* (1), 46-54

Shulamith Lala Ashenberg Straussner
Christine Huff Fewell
New York, NY

A Family Perspective for Substance Abuse: Implications from the Literature

Kenneth J. Gruber
Melissa Floyd Taylor

SUMMARY. This paper calls for researchers and treatment providers to increase their recognition of the role that family and family functioning has for understanding the incidence and impact of substance abuse. Substance abuse is identified as a family problem by exploring its occurrence within families as well as its impact on marital relationship, family violence, and child abuse and neglect. The impact of substance abuse on the roles of spouses and parents are examined, as is the impact of substance abuse on children at various developmental stages. The role of the family as participant in active substance abuse as well as a valuable treatment resource is also explored. Finally, the authors present recommendations for increasing the focus on family in substance abuse research. *[Article copies available for a fee from The Haworth Document Delivery Service: 1-800-HAWORTH. E-mail address: <docdelivery@haworthpress. com> Website: <http://www.HaworthPress.com> © 2006 by The Haworth Press, Inc. All rights reserved.]*

Kenneth J. Gruber, PhD, is Research and Statistical Services Coordinator, School of Human Environmental Sciences, University of North Carolina, Greensboro, P.O. Box 26170, Greensboro, NC 27402-6170 (E-mail: kjgruber@uncg.edu).

Melissa Floyd Taylor, PhD, LCSW, is Assistant Professor, Department of Social Work, University of North Carolina, Greensboro, P.O. Box 26170, Greensboro, NC 27402-6170 (E-mail: mftaylo2@uncg.edu).

[Haworth co-indexing entry note]: "A Family Perspective for Substance Abuse: Implications from the Literature." Gruber, Kenneth J., and Melissa Floyd Taylor. Co-published simultaneously in *Journal of Social Work Practice in the Addictions* (The Haworth Press, Inc.) Vol. 6, No. 1/2, 2006, pp. 1-29; and: *Impact of Substance Abuse on Children and Families: Research and Practice Implications* (ed: Shulamith Lala Ashenberg Straussner, and Christine Huff Fewell) The Haworth Press, Inc., 2006, pp. 1-29. Single or multiple copies of this article are available for a fee from The Haworth Document Delivery Service [1-800-HAWORTH, 9:00 a.m. - 5:00 p.m. (EST). E-mail address: docdelivery@haworthpress.com].

Available online at http://www.haworthpress.com/web/JSWPA
© 2006 by The Haworth Press, Inc. All rights reserved.
doi:10.1300/J160v06n01_01

1

KEYWORDS: Family and substance abuse, impact of family, parental alcohol and drug use, review of literature

INTRODUCTION

While substance abuse has historically been seen as a problem of the individual, substance abuse frequently affects the entire family. Despite the stereotype of the "loner" alcoholic or drug addict, the vast majority of substance abusers (male and female) live in family settings (Wynne et al., 1996). Additionally, most of those who are under the age of 35 either live with, or have at least weekly contact with one or both parents (Stanton & Shadish, 1997). As a consequence it is important to consider how the role of family and the relationship to family relates to the incidence and occurrence of substance abuse.

The importance of considering the impact of substance abuse from a family perspective is supported by numerous examples. One example is the importance that family often plays in affecting the initiation of alcohol or other drug use, the intensity of that use, and the choice of substances. The decision to use or abstain is often dependent on an individual's relationship status with the family, the family coping mechanisms, and other family members' substance use. Another example of family import is the extent to which the family serves as a protective factor or buffer against substance use and its deleterious effects. In families where alcohol and other drugs are disapproved, family members are less inclined to use them. A third example is the effects that the abuse of alcohol and other drugs often has on family members and their relationships with, and behavior towards, the family. Substance use is frequently associated with child abuse and domestic violence. It also is a leading contributor to marital dissatisfaction, family break-ups, and rejection of family members. The importance of the family in understanding alcohol and drug use and abuse is underlined by these highly destructive consequences of alcoholism and drug dependency on the abuser and the family (Gutierres, Russo, & Urbanski, 1994; McCrady, Epstein, & Kahler, 1998).

In an editorial, Copello and Orford (2002) argued that the literature strongly suggests that families are important stakeholders who both aid the process of change and benefit from the improvement of an addiction problem. They concluded that there are considerable benefits to acknowledging and capitalizing on the role of families with respect to getting substance abusers into treatment, maintaining their participation, improving their substance use related outcomes, and reducing negative impact and harm to the family including children. Their conclusion is tempered, however, by the fact that barriers to the extension of treatment to routinely and specifically involve family members still exist. The majority of addiction services remain primarily focused on the individual drinker or drug user while family members and other support network members are involved only peripherally in treatment. They also suggested that because of this emphasis, research efforts are usually focused primarily on the substance user and not on the potentially important outcomes resulting from family involvement.

This paper extends Copello and Orford's thesis by reviewing the literature that shows the roles that families play in the incidence and prevalence of substance abuse. The review of the literature presented here focuses on four key points: substance abuse is a problem for families because: (1) It *occurs* in families, (2) It *harms* families, (3) Families both participate in and can *perpetuate active* addiction, and (4) Families are a potential *treatment and recovery resource*. We wish to note that the review of the literature included in this paper does not extensively include information on the forms or stages of family and the active *treatment* of addiction, but rather focuses on research that explores the impact and effects of substance abuse on the family and its members. Further, the research literature on the role of family and substance abuse has tended to focus largely on parent and child/adolescent issues, and less on other family relations and structures such as mature families, families without children, or other evolving family forms. In recognition of this more inclusive sense of family, at the conclusion of this paper we offer specific recommendations for future research that consider the family beyond the structure and role of parenting of children and adolescents, but one that looks at the family as an essential foundation for understanding substance abuse.

HOW SUBSTANCE ABUSE OCCURS IN FAMILIES

Incidence and Prevalence

Alcoholism is most prevalent in the age group of 18-44, when many individuals are getting married and having families. The National Household Survey on Drug Abuse (NHSDA), conducted in 2000 and 2001, found that 20.5% of those 12 and over reported binge drinking (defined as more than 5 drinks on at least one occasion during the past

30 days). An additional 5.7 % (or 12.9 million people) reported heavy drinking (defined as 5 or more drinks on the same occasion more than 5 days in the past 30 days). An estimated 7.1% of the population, or 15.9 million people over the age of 12 reported the use of an illicit drug within a month of the interview (SAMHSA, 2001). Half of the women who report using drugs are in the childbearing age group of 15-44 (National Institute of Drug Abuse [NIDA], 1997). In two national surveys (SAMHSA, 2001), 3.7% of pregnant women reported using illicit drugs in the past month, while 12.9 % of pregnant women reported using alcohol and 4.6% reported binging. These rates are much lower compared to those for non-pregnant women (49.8% alcohol use, 20.5% binge drinking) (SAMHSA, 2001).

SAMHSA's Office of Applied Studies, Substance Abuse and Mental Health Statistics Sourcebook (Rouse, 1998) reports that family structure is related to illicit substance use among adolescents (12 -17). Based on data collected between 1991-1993, adolescents in families with both biological parents present were least likely to report substance use (approximately 11%), whereas youths from stepparent or one parent households (approximately 18%) were most likely to use illicit drugs.

Genetics and Family History as Causal Factors of Substance Abuse

While substance abuse is clearly a multi-dimensional phenomenon without a clear "cause," the literature suggests that genetically influenced factors have been found to account for 60% of the variance of risk for an alcohol use disorder, with the remaining 40% thought to be sociocultural and environmental (Shuckit & Smith, 2001).

Although no substance dependent gene has been found, there is evidence that a predisposition towards alcoholism may be passed on from father to son (McGue, 1993). The evidence is less conclusive for a heritable component for alcoholism among women. Other work (e.g., Froehlich & Li, 1993; Gorelick, 1993) suggests a genetic role in determining the brain's response in relation to alcohol dependency and use.

While a familial combination of genetic and environmental factors is contributory, a predisposition to develop an abusive consumption habit does not automatically produce alcoholism, problem drinking, or even alcohol use. Family and other social environmental factors can impede any genetic predisposition to use and/or abuse alcohol (Goodwin, 1985; Jang, Vernon, Livesley, Stein, & Wolf, 2001). Researchers have found that there are other important factors linking substance abuse directly to the family (Grant, 2000; Juliana & Goodman, 1997; McCrady & Epstein, 1995; Steinglass, Bennett, Wolin, & Reiss, 1987). For example, children who grow up with an alcoholic parent are at increased risk of abusing alcohol (Baer, Garmezy, McLaughlin, Pokorny, & Wernick, 1987). Family history is further implicated in McMahon and Luthar's (1998) report of research showing that substance-abusing parents to be more likely themselves to have grown up in chaotic and emotionally problematic family environments: families characterized by psychological maltreatment due to parental neglect, physical or sexual abuse, economic distress, and other family depleting conditions. Moreover, parents from substance abusing homes are more likely to report the parenting styles of their parents as punitive and authoritarian.

Family Environment and Substance Use

The family environment often plays a significant role in the use of alcohol and other drugs. Unstable and inconsistent family and living environment factors (e.g., transient living conditions, inconsistent caretaking, violence) resulting from substance using caretakers have been linked to the incidence of psychological and emotional development problems among their children. In families where alcohol and other drugs are used or attitudes towards their use is positive, the incidence of children's usage is higher than in families where usage is low and where attitudes towards drugs are not as permissive (Brook, Brook, Whiteman, Gordon, & Cohen, 1990; Johnson, Schoutz, and Locke, 1984). Gfroerer (1987) reported that among a sample of adolescents and their older siblings and parents, youths were twice as likely to try marijuana if there was parental or older sibling drug use. Boyd and Holmes (2002) found among a sample of African American women cocaine users that their substance use paralleled use patterns of their family members, particularly those of fathers, uncles, and brothers.

Alcoholism is also less likely to be passed on to offspring among families that maintain family rituals (Wynne et al., 1996), while children from families with one or both alcoholic parents who experience disrupted family rituals surrounding dinner time, evenings, holidays, weekends, vacations, and visitors are more likely themselves to develop alcohol use problems (Wohlin, Bennett, Noonan, & Teitelbaum, 1980).

Family role structures and role assignments can be barriers to facing substance use and abuse issues. Processes relating to management of feelings, role structures communication and need fulfillment within the family system are related to drug abuse behavior (Haber, 2000). For example, in situations in which alcohol-related behaviors have become embedded in family routines, rituals, and problem-solving strategies, changing the alcoholic's drinking status can be challenging for the family (Steinglass et al., 1987).

It has been reported that avoidance of conflict with the drug user can reinforce substance-abusing behavior (McCrady & Epstein, 1995; O'Farrell & Fals-Stewart, 2000). Disapproval and distancing by family members can delay the abuser from confronting addiction and related behaviors (McCrady & Epstein, 1995). Alcohol abuse often is tolerated because it "enables" the abuser to be more emotionally accessible to other family members. As Haber (2000) notes, "family members may become addicted to emotional crises because crises are the only route to getting in touch with and expressing otherwise repressed or suppressed feelings" (p. 316). Ignoring or avoiding alcohol abuse as a problem is often associated with significant distress not only among the immediate family but among relatives as it contributes to family conflict and a negative family climate (Orford et al., 2001).

FAMILIES AND THE PERPETUATION
OF SUBSTANCE ABUSE

Family Climate and Functioning

A functioning family is one that offers an environment that provides for the successful development and protection of its members. This outcome reflects a secure, cohesive, and mutually supportive family environment–one that is characterized by appropriate roles, effective communication, and routine expression of positive affect, and one that is based on a shared set of cultural norms and values. Family members must be emotionally involved with each other and able to influence each other's behavior as it relates to the functioning of the family (Moss, Lynch, Hardie, & Baron, 2002). In the substance affected family, functional family roles are often distorted or missing. For example, children of alcoholic parents may be parentified and take on parenting and adult responsibilities that may preclude them from age appropriate activities or peer group socialization experiences (Haber, 2000).

The family unit can be conceptualized as systems with interdependencies among its members. An implication of this perspective is that when one part of the system changes or is "damaged" it impacts other parts of the system. Another implication is that as a system the family may adapt to protect and accommodate the substance user resulting in accommodating dysfunctional family relationships. This adaptation often includes denial and subterfuge to avoid addressing the issue, and the implementation of family rules and behaviors that mask family member dependency behavior (Stevens-Smith, 1998). Another implication of a systemic perspective is the potential for reciprocal impact of substance use and abuse and other family member behavior. Stewart and Brown (1993), for example, suggest that adolescent problem behavior may be both a cause and a reaction to family drug use. As a consequence, resolution of an adolescent's drug use can lead to better family functioning and improved communication and support for the adolescent.

The onset of substance abuse is frequently associated with stress and may be precipitated by family disruptions, control or management issues, or losses (Bennett, 1995). Accordingly, it has been well established that family members often have a central role in the course of alcohol or drug addiction (Liddle & Dakof, 1995; Margolis & Zweben, 1998; Moore & Finkelstein, 2001; Moos, Finney, & Cronkite, 1990; Noel, Stout, & Malloy, 1993; O'Farrell & Fals-Stewart, 2000) and its treatment (Edwards & Steinglass, 1995; cf. O'Farrell; 1993; Stanton & Shadish, 1997). This role has both negative and positive implications for treatment and outcomes. Problems that may have been masked by substance abuse may become evident when substance abuse is no longer an issue (Haber, 2000). Steinglass and others (Steinglass et al., 1987) found that the status of alcohol use (abuse, transition to recovery, recovery) affects family interaction patterns and their adaptive responses to situations and conditions associated with the family's use status.

Substance-Affected Spouses. Alcohol abuse has been shown to be both a precipitant and consequence of marital stress, spousal abuse, and separation and divorce (Amato & Previti, 2003; Halford & Osgarby, 1993; Wilsnack, 1996). Stressful marital interactions are associated with exacerbation of alcohol abuse and failed abstinence (Halford & Osgarby, 1993; Kahler, McCrady, & Epstein, 2003). Substance abusers often marry or partner with other substance abusers (McCrady & Epstein, 1995). Research indicates that discrepancy in substance use by couples is related to lower marital quality and higher marital stress (Fals-Stewart, Birchler, & O'Farrell, 1999; Mudar, Leonard, & Soltysinski, 2001; Wilsnack & Wilsnack, 1993). Alcohol abuse is related to separation and divorce, though it may be as much of a consequence as it is a predictor of the dissolution of a marital relationship. Encouragingly, for some, marriage and parenthood may also serve as a transition point for terminating drug abuse (Yamaguchi & Kandel, 1985).

Research supports the contention that stressful spousal or partner relationships can trigger the desire to return to or continue the abuse of alcohol and other drugs (Sullivan, Wolk, & Hartmann, 1992). Poor communication and problem-solving, arguing, financial stressors, and nagging are often reported as antecedents to drug abuse. Resentment by the abuser towards efforts to intervene or control substance abuse behavior sometimes serves as a cue to continue consumption (Wynne et al., 1996). Among drinking spouses, mismatched drinking patterns (one spouse drinking more or more frequently than the other) can indicate distress or conflict in the relationship. Husbands and boyfriends are more likely to deny that their spouse or partner has a drinking problem or is in need of treatment (McCrady et al., 1998; Wilsnack, 1996).

Most spouses attempt to get their alcohol abusing partners to reduce their drinking through aversive techniques such as nagging, complaining and threatening (Thomas & Ager, 1993). These efforts are typically implemented on an occasional or unsystematic basis and generally are not effective–resulting in negative abuser reactions and exacerbation of existing marital conflict and disagreement. These negative consequences may serve to exacerbate the problem, resulting in the abuser leaving home to drink or imbibe secretly (McCrady & Epstein, 1995; McCrady et al., 1998).

Substance-Affected Parents. The family environments of drug using parents are frequently characterized as being chaotic with frequent residence changes, minimal contacts with fathers, and severe shortages of financial resources for the basic necessities and needs of the children. Often, social support is also limited or nonexistent due to the disorganization and instability of these families (Harden, 1998).

Many parents addicted to drugs have not experienced positive parenting models and often themselves feel inadequate as parents. Despite these feelings, many substance affected parents want to be good parents, but need specific training to overcome their inadequacies and issues related to their alcohol and other drug use (Juliana & Goodman, 1997). To the extent substance abuse impairs a parent's ability to parent, chemical dependency can have serious consequences for a child and for the parent to fulfill her/his role as a positive role model and primary caregiver (Harden, 1998; Murray, 1989). Adding to the problem, parents with substance abuse problems often experience social isolation and marginalization. They are often absent parents (Kumpfer, 1987) due to incapacitation from drug or alcohol use, or due to time spent in procuring substances, being in treatment, or in jail or prison (Dunn, Tarter, Mezzich, Vanyukov, Kirisci, & Kirillova, 2002).

Parental substance abuse is often associated with family dysfunction and the risk of abusive parenting behavior, including child abuse and neglect (Chaffin, Kelleher, & Hollenberg, 1996; Hampton, Senatore, & Gullota, 1998; Hien & Honeyman, 2000). There is also evidence to suggest that drug use may magnify a parent's *incapacity* to parent, leading to more problematic parent-child relationships (Hans, Bernstein, & Henson, 1999). Comorbidity of substance use and mental disorders also has been widely documented: Depression, bi-polar illness, and generalized anxiety disorders have all been found to be associated with problematic parenting and substance use (Bays, 1990; Luthar, Merakangas, & Rounsaville, 1993).

Parenting styles and behaviors have been related to both the onset and development of substance abuse among children and adolescents. Parent-youth conflict, harsh parenting (involving severe physical punishment or verbal reprimand), poor monitoring, ineffective control, permissiveness, and lack of parental warmth all have been related to substance abuse by youth (Griffin, Botvin, Scheier, Diaz, & Miller, 2000; Kumpfer, Alvarado, & Whiteside, 2003; Lochman & Steenhoven, 2002; McGillicuddy, Rychtarik, Duquette, & Morsheimer, 2001; Webb, Bray, Getz, & Adams, 2002). Research also suggests that mothers' and fathers' different parenting styles have differential effects on their children's propensity to use drugs (Baumrind, 1991).

Substance-Affected Mothers. Substance affected women report more guilt and shame and more conflict over their marital and parental roles (Kahler et al., 2003), and are often worried about losing legal and physical custody of their children. Substance dependent mothers often report feeling ineffective and incompetent as parents, experience low bonding with their babies, and perceive them as overly demanding (Davis, 1994; Kelley, 1992). Feelings of inadequacy as mothers and perceptions of rejection by their infants leads some substance using mothers to increase their drug use in order to cope. The absence of involved fathers is a common characteristic of children being raised by substance abusing mothers (Davis, 1994), and, at times, the children may be abandoned by their drug dependent mothers.

It is important to note that substance abuse by mothers does not *always* equal poor parenting (Baker & Carson, 1999). Suchman and Luthar (2000), for example, found that the only parenting factor directly related to maternal addiction was lack of sufficient parental involvement, while other parenting factors, such as control over autonomy and limit-setting, may be better explained by determinants other than substance abuse. There is, however, considerable evidence that links poor parenting with substance and alcohol use. Maternal drug addiction has been unequivocally linked with parenting deficits, including harmful parenting styles, discipline, intolerance of child behavior, and insensitivity to both children's needs and stage-specific development issues (Suchman & Luthar, 2000). Maternal substance abuse has also been found to have serious developmental implications for children (Brooks, Zuckerman, Bamforth, Cole, & Kaplan-Sanoff, 1994). Prenatal drug exposure is associated with increased levels of parenting stress and child maltreatment. Recent research has shown that there is an increasing prevalence of alcohol consumption among pregnant women (Ebrahim, Luman, Floyd, Murphy, Bennett, & Boyle, 1998).

Chemically dependent women often display ineffective parenting skills and practices related to childrearing (Davis, 1994; Fiks, Johnson, & Rosen, 1985). Drug abuse has also been found to be associated with higher potential for punitiveness and greater severity in maternal disciplinary practices (Hien & Honeyman, 2000; Miller, Smyth, & Mudar, 1999). In some cases, the lifestyles of drug using mothers are incongruent with adequate parenting (Harden, 1998). Women involved in deviant or criminal activities, such as prostitution or selling illegal drugs, are likely to have serious deficits in their capacity to provide for the emotional and developmental needs of their children. Moreover, exposure to violence and other negative life events can reduce their ability to properly supervise and interact with their children.

Substance-Affected Fathers. The role of substance-affected fathering in the family has not been as adequately explored as that of substance-affected mothering. McMahon and Rounsaville (2002) call for the inclusion of fathers in the substance abuse research agenda. Absent, substance-abusing fathers have been implicated in what had been previously thought to be maternal effects of substance abuse on urban children (Frank, Brown, Johnson, & Cabral, 2002). Paternal alcoholism has been associated with heightened sensitivity and lower tolerance to the behaviors and needs of their infant children (Eiden, Chavez, & Leonard, 1999; Eiden & Leonard, 2000). Noll, Zucker, Fitzgerald, and Curtis (1992), for example, found that male preschoolers with alcoholic fathers had significantly less advanced personal and social development than controls. Cognitive development has also been found to be impacted by paternal alcohol problems. Finally, some research suggests that drinking by fathers directly affects adolescent drinking, but mothers' drinking is not predictive of youths' use of alcohol (Zhang, Welte, & Wieczorek, 1999).

Siblings. Older siblings are a source of drugs and often use drugs with their younger siblings (Needle, McCubbin, Wilson, Reineck, Lazar, & Mederer, 1986). Brook, Whiteman, Gordon, and Brook (1988) found that older brother use and advocacy of use of drugs was associated with their younger brothers' use. Studies have noted that sibling use may be a more powerful indicator of sibling substance use than either parental use or parents' attitudes towards drug use (Needle et al., 1986).

Extended Family Members. It bears mentioning that in this era of evolving family forms, extended family members are also affected by substance abuse. There appears to be some evidence that extended family members, or second-degree relatives, both impact the nuclear family through substance abuse and are similarly impacted by substance abuse in the nuclear family (Orford, Dalton, Hartney, Ferrins-Brown, Kerr, & Maslin, 2002; Ragin, Pilotti, Madry, Sage, Bingham, & Primm, 2002).

HOW SUBSTANCE ABUSE HARMS FAMILIES

Substance abuse in families is frequently accompanied by other problems, such as mental illness, domestic violence, economic difficulties, housing needs, and residence in dangerous neighborhood environments (Semidei, Radel, & Nolan, 2001). Substance abusing families tend to be characterized by low levels of cohesion, low frustration tolerance, unrealistic expectations of children, role reversal, isolation, and poor parenting skills–characteristics associated with adverse consequences for families (Johnson & Leff, 1999; Sheridan, 1995). Substance abuse has also been related to destructive family behaviors, including child abuse and neglect (Bays, 1990; Davis, 1994; Famularo, Kinscherff, & Fenton, 1992; Sheridan, 1995) and incest (Hurley, 1991).

Child Abuse and Neglect

Studies of samples of child abuse cases have frequently shown that parental substance use is associated with child maltreatment (Ammerman, Kolko, Kirisci, Blackson, & Dawes, 1999; Kelly, 1992; Dore, Doris & Wright, 1995; Dunn et al., 2002; Magura & Laudet, 1996; Sheridan, 1995). Moreover, child abuse *potential* may be increased when a parent is affected by a substance abuse disorder (Ammerman et al., 1999). Parental stress and low frustration tolerance are often cited as a reason for child abuse and neglect, but other factors such as inadequate parenting skills, social isolation, and the behavior of the children are likely contributors to substance affected parents' physical and emotional abuse and neglect of their children (Ammerman et al., 1999; Kelley, 1992). Families affected by substance abuse are prone to be conflicted and abusive leading to less effort towards and opportunities for effective parenting (Dunn et al., 2002).

Out of Home Placement. Parental neglect and abuse related to substance abuse is a frequently cited reason for removing children from their parents (Azzi-Lessing & Olsen, 1996; Famularo et al., 1992; Kelley, 1992).

Family Violence

The frequent co-occurrence of substance abuse and family violence is well documented. Substance abuse is well identified as an important risk factor for family violence, particularly in cases involving serious violence, including homicide (Brookoff, O'Brien, Cook, Thompson, & Williams, 1997; Easton, Swan, & Sinha, 2000). Alcoholism and other substance abuse have been shown to be related to partner aggression (Bennett, Tolman, Rogalski, & Srinivasaraghavan, 1994; Kahler, McCrady, & Epstein, 2003; Kantor & Straus, 1989; Stuart, Moore, Ramsey, & Kahler, 2003). Hotaling and Sugarman (1986) reviewed 52 studies addressing husband-to-wife violence and found alcohol use was one of four consistent risk markers characterizing violent husbands. Other studies have found that the severity of substance abuse is related to the extent of conjugal violence (Brown, Werk, Caplan, & Seraganian, 1999; Brown, Werk, Caplan, Shields, & Seraganian, 1998).

SUBSTANCE-AFFECTED CHILDREN

Children are perhaps those *most* affected by substance abuse in the family. One widely cited estimate suggests that one in four children in the United States under the age 18 is exposed to alcohol abuse or dependence in their family (Grant, 2000). There is clear evidence that children of parents who abuse alcohol or other drugs are at measurable risk for developing emotional behavioral and/or social problems (Grant, 2000; Kelley & Fals-Stewart, 2002). Clinical studies have shown that children of alcoholics are more likely to be diagnosed with a childhood psychiatric disorder than children of nonalcoholic parents (Moss, Mezzich, Yao, Gavaler, & Martin, 1995, West & Prinz, 1987). The likelihood of having adverse childhood experiences is higher for children growing up in homes where one parent was alcoholic, and *highest* for those growing up in households where *both* parents were alcoholic (Dube, Anda, Felitti, Croft, Edwards, & Giles, 2001).

Parental abuse of alcohol and other drugs can have a significant negative impact on a child. Young children may experience considerable difficulty comprehending changes in their parents' temperament or behavior when affected by alcohol and other drugs. In addition to possible social humiliation and shame a child may experience as the result of public exposure of their parent's substance abuse or its effects, such use, particularly involving illicit drugs, may lead to involvement in and negative consequences from law enforcement and other branches of the judicial system. The emotional impact of parental substance abuse also may be significant. Children may experience anger, anxiety, or fear about their parents and about what will happen to them. Fear of abandonment, helplessness, hopelessness, and even guilt over not interceding to prevent their parent's alcohol or drug uses are not uncommon among latency age children (Dore, Kauffman, & Nelson-Zlupko, 1996; Murray, 1989).

Children who grow up with an alcoholic parent are susceptible to psychological, behavioral, and school problems (Moos, Finney, & Cronkite, 1990). Studies have shown that parental alcohol abuse has been related to childhood psychopathology (West & Prinz, 1987) and adjustment problems in young adults (Clair & Genest, 1987; Felitti et al., 1998). Parent relapse has negative effects on children's physical and social functioning (Moos, Finney, & Cronkite, 1990). Children who grow up in substance-abusing dysfunctional families often learn maladaptive role expectations that impair their relationships later in life. They have unrealistic expectations of themselves, difficulty with accepting authority and problems with intimacy, trust, and emotional balance (Craig, 1993).

Murray (1989) noted that parental alcoholism is probably disruptive to family life, but measuring the disruption and linking it to specific behavior is problematic. Children's vulnerability to their parent's behavior and the impact of substance abuse on them is likely dependent on a complex of social and environmental factors and the child's specific stage of development.

Impact on Early Child Development

Recent research indicates that as many 10% of newborns have been exposed to alcohol or drugs (Azmitia, 2001). Earlier statistics estimated that prenatal exposure to drugs ranges from 350,000 (Chasnoff, 1989) to 739,200 (Center for the Future of Children, 1991). Alarmingly, the incidence of fetal alcohol syndrome (FAS) and alcohol-related neurodevelopmental disorder (ARND) has been estimated to be at least 9.1 of every 1,000 births, or nearly one in every 100 live births (Sampson et al., 1997). In fact, FAS is the number one cause of mental retardation in children (Azmitia, 2001).

Deficient growth, abnormal brain development, neurobehavioral impairments, and sensory and sensory-motor defects have all been linked to prenatal maternal drug use (Chasnoff & Lowder, 1999; Dunn et al., 2002; Greenberg, 1999, 2000). Prenatal cocaine use, for example, has been directly linked to low developmental scores at birth (Behnke, Eyler, Garvan, Wobie, & Hou, 2002).

Prenatal exposure to alcohol and other drugs is widely seen as a harmful influence on children's later development (Harden, 1998; Johnson & Leff, 1999). Prenatal alcohol and marijuana exposure, for example, has also been found to adversely impact learning and memory skills in 10 year olds (Richardson, Ryan, Willford, Day, & Goldschmidt, 2002). Additional studies have found similar cognitive problems (McNichol & Tash, 2001). Hawley, Halle, Drasin, and Thomas (1995) found that problems related to cognitive, language, and emotional development of children were higher among children of cocaine addicted mothers.

Again, although various studies have found relationships between parental alcohol abuse and negative development in children (e.g., see Johnson & Leff, 1999), it is not clear whether these and other developmental effects are directly related to early effects of substance abuse–such as altered brain chemistry (Azmitia, 2001)–or to effects of inadequate parenting and nurturing, or other social and developmental factors (Hans, 2002). For some children, it is the fact that they may be "parentified" early in life by having to take care of a "sick" parent that deprives them of a "normal" path of development and consequent psychological and behavioral reactions (Murray, 1989).

Early Childhood/Latency Age Children

The impact of parental alcoholism on young children includes conduct problems, depression, anxiety, hyperactivity, low self-esteem, peer aggression, poor school performance, and reduced sense of self-efficacy (Dore et al., 1996). The impact of parental substance abuse on cognitive functioning, as it manifests in academic performance may be related to deficits in parent supervision and schoolwork monitoring.

Adolescents

Considerable evidence exists to suggest that both parental substance use and attitudes towards drug use are major factors affecting substance use among adolescents (Baer, Garmezy, McLaughlin, Pokorny, & Wernick, 1987; Brook, Brook, Whiteman, Gordon, & Cohen, 1990; Chassin, Curran, Hussong, & Colder, 1999; Li, Pentz, & Chou, 2002; Thompson & Wilsnick, 1987). By contrast, non-use of substances by parents has been identified as serving a buffering function in protecting adolescents from using alcohol and other drugs (Li, Pentz, & Chou, 2002).

Parent-adolescent conflict has been strongly associated with youth involvement with alcohol and other drugs (Baer et al. 1987; Hops, Tildesley, Lichestein, Ary, & Sherman, 1990). Adolescents use alcohol and other drugs to ease tension at home or to show rebellion against parental authority (Thompson & Wilsnack, 1987). On the other hand, positive family relations including parental affection and support have been found to be a deterrent to adolescent drug use (Bowser & Word, 1993; Stewart & Brown, 1993). Brook, Brook, Whiteman, Gordon, and Cohen (1990) found that adolescent drug use is inversely correlated with parent-adolescent attachment, which includes parental involvement in limit setting, parental assertiveness, affection and child-centeredness, and identification of children with parents.

Adults Children of Substance Abusers

The effects of family substance use and abuse on children do not end once children grow up. As the research on adult children of alcoholics (COAs) shows, many remain at risk for behavioral, psychological, cognitive, and neuropsychological deficits well into adulthood (Anda et al., 2002; Chassin, Pitts, DeLucia, & Todd, 1999; Johnson & Leff, 1999; Scharff, Broida, Conway, & Yue, 2004). Specifically, COAs may experience long-term impairment in self-esteem regulation, the maintenance of intimate relationships (Lewchanin & Sweeney, 1997) and increased feelings of shame (Hawkins, 1996).

FAMILIES AS A TREATMENT AND RECOVERY RESOURCE

The need to address family issues in a comprehensive treatment program is becoming widely recognized (Craig, 1993; Kelley & Fals-Stewart, 2002; McIntyre, 2004; Straussner, 2004). Family involvement is often sought because of the critical role it has in getting addicts into treatment, participating in aftercare, and preventing relapse and maintaining recovery (Costantini, Wermuth, Sorenson, & Lyons, 1992; Gruber & Fleetwood, 2004; Gruber, Fleetwood, & Harding, 2001; Knight & Simpson, 1996; Margolis & Zweben, 1998; McCrady et al., 1998; Ossip-Klein & Rychtarik, 1993; Stevens-Smith, 1998).

The literature shows that parent and family oriented intervention programs can be effective in preventing and reducing youth substance abuse (Lochman & Steenhoven, 2002). Women who report support from partners or spouses are more likely to remain in treatment (Knight, Hood, Logan, & Chatham, 1999) and to have better treatment outcomes (Gutierres, Russo, & Urbanski, 1994; Weiss, Martinez-Raga, Griffin, Greenfield, & Hufford, 1997).

FAMILIES AS A PREVENTIVE RESOURCE: RISK AND RESILIENCY

The concepts of "risk and resiliency" are important factors to consider in the treatment and prevention of alcohol and other drug use (McCubbin, McCubbin,Thompson, & Han, 1999). Risk refers to the confluence of factors that relate to the probability of an individual's chemical use and dependence. Resiliency refers to the capability of an individual to avoid or recover from adverse effects of alcohol or drug use. When related to families, the determination of risk and resiliency is much more complex, but nevertheless important to achieving either avoidance or minimizing the negative effects of substance abuse on the individual and the family. Family risk (and conversely resiliency or protective factors) is more than just the summation of risk for individual family members. Rather it involves what family members bring to the family dynamics, its processes, and its determination of the family unit (McCubbin, McCubbin, Thompson, & Han, 1999).

There has been increased attention in targeting family resilience factors in reducing the onset and frequency of adolescent substance abuse. The presumption is that by increasing family action factors, such as bonding in the family, involvement of the family in community activities with their children, and use of community services to address family or youth problems, substance use among youths can be reduced or avoided (Johnson, Bryant, Collins, Noe, Strader, & Berbaum, 1998). Hawkins, Catalano, and Miller (1992) in a review of risk and protective factors for alcohol and other drug problems in adolescence and early adulthood concluded that family and family environment related factors, such as (a) family alcohol and drug use and attitudes toward/ permissiveness of use, (b) family behavior and activity management practices, (c) family conflict, and (d) low family bonding, contributed to youth substance use. Conversely, they identified protective family and family environment factors to include: (a) high family bonding and parental attachment, (b) stable family environments, and (c) supportive family environments.

The means by which family characteristics might serve as protective factors, at least for children and adolescents, are suggested by Brooks and others (e.g., Brooks et al., 1994). They suggest that parental attachment, positive role modeling, and vigilant monitoring resulting in compensatory actions by parents to intervene may reduce youth initiation in or patterns of use of substances that result in problematic drug or alcohol use. Interventions that focus on protective factor development through improvement of parenting and family functioning have been able to show positive results in improvements in children's social and emotional functioning (Atkan, Kumfer, & Turner, 1996) and reduction in anti-social behavior linked to adolescence substance use (Hogue, Liddle, Becker, & Johnson-Leckrone, 2002).

CONCLUSIONS

The literature reviewed in this paper underscores the fact that substance abuse occurs in families, harms families, and that families are important to both the etiology of addiction and recovery. Our assessment of the state of the literature suggests that a more comprehensive inclusion of families in future studies warrants consideration. To this end, we conclude our paper with recommendations for strengthening the family perspective in six areas of substance abuse research and treatment.

1. *Incidence, prevalence, and impact of substance abuse.*

Because most studies count the incidence, prevalence, and impact of substance abuse in terms of the individual substance abuser, it is simply not determinable to what extent families are negatively impacted by alcohol and other drug abuse by a family member. Studies of child abuse, neglect, and domestic violence have linked substance abuse to the occurrence of these events. Studies of children of alcoholics also suggest that there may be long-term negative effects of growing up in a substance abusing family, including intergenerational substance abuse, adult adjustment problems, especially in the area of intimate relationships, and a general inability to move beyond the early adverse experiences. In the future, it will be essential to expand and modify current methods of assessing incidence and prevalence in order to capture the family *as a whole.*

2. *Substance abuse as related to the functional characteristics of the family.*

There is a need for a change in *philosophical stance* that both honors the richness and dynamic nature of families and at the same time, illuminates points of inquiry that reflect this stance. For example, when families are considered in substance abuse research and treatment, it often is from a "snapshot view" or a picture of the family frozen in time. In other words, dynamic families with rich histories are reduced in many ways to one "treatment episode" or seen only in relation to their effect on the substance abuser. What is missing are the ways in which substance abuse impacts the factors that make families, well . . . families. In particular, it is important to know how the functional characteristics–relationships, responsibilities, alliances, roles, rules, and behavior–of families all contribute to the impact that substance abuse has on the family. Consequently, in order to improve our understanding of substance abuse as both a determinant of poor family functioning and as a consequence of family dysfunction, it is essential to develop more systematic inquiries into these functional characteristics and relationships (Csiernik, 2002).

3. *Developmental stages of family substance abuse and recovery.*

Substance use in families is not a static occurrence but is likely to follow a developmental pathway from experimentation to misuse to abuse or dependency. Problematic use along this continuum may follow a number of paths that reflect stages of improvement or recovery (e.g., see Brown & Lewis, 1999; Carboni & DiClemente, 2000; Connors, Donovan, & DiClemente, 2001). But, just as substance abuse changes, families change as well and the impact of the substance abusing family member may have minor to moderate impact on the family. Important too, is the composition of the family (i.e., young versus older children) and the availability of support within and outside the family to address the impact that the abuse of alcohol and other drugs has had (Straussner, 2004).

To increase our understanding and the development of more effective interventions, more research needs to focus on the impact on substance abuse in families *over time,* and not just during isolated contacts with treatment providers. It is essential to factor in the developmental aspects of substance use as well as the developmental path of factors such as social capital (Granfield & Cloud, 2001) that relate to recovery to better determine what is needed to be done in cases where it occurs. Understanding family involvement in recovery efforts along a continuum based on the substance abuser's level of motivation is another way of taking developmental factors into account (Thomas & Corcoran, 2001).

4. *Families as the unit of measurement in the study of substance abuse.*

The primary assumption of this paper is that the family is a critical point of consideration for addressing most cases of substance dependency. Consequently, instead of isolating individuals within families we need to develop ways to look at the effects of addictions on the entire family. Though many studies have included assessments of spouses, parents, children, and in some cases other family members, the vast majority of studies have not considered the substance-affected client as part of the family that includes these individuals and the multiple family roles that they may fulfill. For example, an adult male may be a father, spouse, and child (to his parents)–and these family membership categories have different implications for the family and for how substance abuse affects the roles and responsibilities associated with each of these roles. Therefore, it is critical to consider the impact a family member may have as a function of multiple roles and their impact on different family function characteristics.

5. *Families as resources for developing strategies to combat alcohol and drug addiction.*

It is well documented that parents are important models for their children's substance use (e.g., see Lyter & Lyter, 2003). Parents who use alcohol and drugs often raise children who also use alcohol and drugs. It is also frequently the case that in couples in which one member has an alcohol or drug problem, the non-using partner will develop a substance use problem or co-dependency to keep the couple together. These "sources of influence" represent potential keys for the developing of effective prevention and intervention strategies, by virtue of their "association" on a variety of social, emotional, and physical levels. These levels in turn impact a variety of influence processes such as modeling, socialization, behavior modification, and the deterioration of emotional boundaries. Therefore, the connections among family members represents a rich source for investigating some of the major pathways by which many individuals become exposed and ultimately dependent on alcohol and other drugs. This is especially important as we have historically underestimated the *positive* influence that families can exert upon members struggling with addiction (see Thomas & Corcoran, 2001).

6. *Family risk and protective factors related to substance abuse.*

A final line of recommended inquiry is family-related risk and protective factors as moderators or mediators of problematic behavior (e.g., see Hawkins, Catalano, & Miller, 1992). This perspective has been primarily examined with respect to child and adolescent substance abuse (Lyter & Lyter, 2003), and it is time to extend this view to families. Because families are dynamic entities changing throughout its cycle of development, a risk and protective factors perspective is well equipped to capture changes in the family's barriers and resources to positive family functioning and relationships. Finally, by moving to a risk and protection focus, there is less of an emphasis on family pathology and more emphasis on avenues of recovery–a perspective that benefits all family members.

REFERENCES

Aktan, G.B., Kumpfer, K.L., & Turner, C.W. (1996). Effectiveness of a family skills training program for substance use prevention with inner city African-American families. *Substance Use & Misuse, 31,* 157-175.

Amato, P.R., & Previti, D. (2003). People's reasons for divorcing: Gender, social class, the life course, and adjustment. *Journal of Family Issues, 24*(5), 602-626.

Ammerman, R.T., Kolko, D. J., Kirisci, L., Blackson, T.C., & Dawes, M.A. (1999). Child abuse potential in parents with histories of substance use disorder. *Child Abuse & Neglect, 23*(12), 1225-1238.

Anda, R.F., Whitfield, C.L., Felitti, V.J., Chapman, D., Edwards, V.J., Dube, S.R., & Williamson, D.F. (2002). Adverse childhood experiences, alcoholic parents, and later risk of alcoholism and depression. *Psychiatric Services, 53*(8), 1001-1009.

Azmitia, E. C. (2001). Impact of drugs and alcohol on the brain through the life cycle: Knowledge for social workers. *Journal of Social Work Practice in the Addictions, 1*(3), 41-64.

Azzi-Lessing, L., & Olsen, L.J. (1996). Substance abuse-affected families in the child welfare system: New challenges, new alliances. *Social Work, 41,* 15-23.

Baer, P.E., Garmezy, L.B., McLaughlin, R.J., Pokorny, A.D., & Wernick, M.J. (1987). Stress coping, family conflict, and adolescent alcohol use. *Journal of Behavioral Medicine, 10,* 449-466.

Baker, P. L., & Carson, A. (1999). "I take care of my kids" Mothering practices of substance-abusing women. *Gender & Society, 13*(3), 347-363.

Barnes, G.M., & Welte, J.W. (1990). Prediction of adult's drinking patterns from the drinking of their parents. *Journal of Studies on Alcohol, 51*(6), 523-527.

Baumrind, D. (1991). The influence of parenting style on adolescent competence and substance abuse. *Journal of Early Adolescence, 11*(1), 56-95.

Bays, J. (1990). Substance abuse and child abuse: Impact of addiction on the child. *Pediatric Clinics of North America, 37(4),* 881-904.

Behnke, M., Eyler, F.D., Garavan, C.W., Wobie, K., & Hou, W. (2002). Cocaine exposure and developmental outcome from birth to 6 months. *Neurotoxicology & Teratology, 24*(3), 283-295.

Bennett, L.W. (1995). Substance abuse and the domestic assault of women. *Social Work, 40*(6), 760-771.

Bennett, L.W., Tolman, R. M., Rogalski, C.J., & Srinivasaraghavan, J. (1994). Domestic abuse by male alcohol and drug addicts. *Violence and Victims, 9,* 359-368.

Bowser, B.P., & Word, C.O. (1993). Comparison of African-American adolescent crack cocaine users and nonusers: Background factors in drug use and HIV sexual risk behaviors. *Psychology of Addictive Behaviors, 7*(3), 155-161.

Boyd, C.J., & Holmes, C. (2002). Women who smoke crack and their family substance abuse problems. *Health Care for Women International, 23, 576-586.*

Brook, J.S., Brook, D.W., Whiteman, M., Gordon, A.S., & Cohen, P. (1990). The psychosocial etiology of adolescent drug use: A family interactional approach. *Genetic, Social & General Psychology Monographs, 116* (2), 112 -267.

Brookoff, D., O'Brien, K.K., Cook, C.S., Thompson, T.D., & Williams, C. (1997). Characteristics of participants in domestic violence. *Journal of the American Medical Association, 277,* 1369-1373.

Brooks, C.S., Zuckerman, B., Bamforth, A., Cole, J., & Kaplan-Sanoff, M. (1994). Clinical issues related to substance-involved mothers and their infants. *Infant Mental Health Journal 15*(2), 202-217.

Brown, S., & Lewis, V. (1999). *The alcoholic family in recovery: A developmental model.* New York: The Guilford Press.

Brown, T.G., Werk, A., Caplan, T., & Seraganian, P. (1999). Violent substance abusers in domestic violence treatment. *Violence and Victims, 14,* 179-190.

Brown, T.G., Werk, A., Caplan, T., Shields, N., & Seraganian, P. (1998). Incidence and characteristics of violent men in substance abuse treatment. *Addictive Behaviors, 23,* 573-586.

Carboni, J.P., & DiClemente, C.C. (2000). Using transtheoretical model profiles to differentiate levels of alcohol abstinence success. *Journal of Consulting & Clinical Psychology, 68,* 810-817.

Chassin, L., Curran, P.J., Hussong, A.M., & Colder, C.R. (1996). The relation of parental alcoholism to adolescent substance use: A longitudinal follow-up study. *Journal of Abnormal Psychology, 105*(1), 70-80.

Chassin, L., Pitts, S.C., DeLucia, C., & Todd, M. (1999). A longitudinal study of children of alcoholics predicting young adult substance use disorders, anxiety, and depression. *Journal of Abnormal Psychology, 108*(1), 106-119.

Clair, D. J., & Genest, M. (1987). Variables associated with the adjustment of offspring of alcoholic fathers. *Journal of Studies on Alcohol, 48,* 345-355.

Connors, G. J., Donovan, D.M., & DiClemente, C.C. (2001). *Substance abuse treatment and stages of change.* New York: The Guilford Press.

Copello, A., & Orford, J. (2002). Addiction and the family: Is it time for services to take notice of the evidence? *Addictions, 97,* 1361-1363.

Costantini, M. F., Wermuth, L., Sorenson, J.L., & Lyons, J.S. (1992). Family functioning as a predictor of progress in substance abuse treatment. *Journal of Substance Abuse Treatment, 9,* 331-335.

Craig, R.J. (1993). Contemporary trends in substance abuse. *Professional Psychology: Research and Practice, 24,* 182-189.

Csiernik, R. (2002). Counseling for the family: The neglected aspect of addiction treatment in Canada. *Social Work Practice in the Addictions* 2(1), 79-92.

Davis, S. (1994). Effects of chemical dependency in parenting women. In R.R. Watson (Ed.), *Drug and alcohol abuse reviews: Addictive behaviors in women (Vol. 5)* (pp. 381-414). Totowa NJ: Humana Press.

Dore, M.M., Doris, J.M., & Wright, P. (1995). Identifying substance abuse in maltreating families: A child welfare challenge. *Child Abuse & Neglect, 19,* 531-543.

Dore, M.M., Kauffman, E., Nelson-Zlupko, L., & Granfort, E. (1996). Psychosocial functioning and treatment needs of latency-age children from drug-involved families. *Families in Society* 77(10), 595-604.

Dube, S. R., Anda, R. F., Felitti, V. J., Croft, J. B., Edwards, V. J., & Giles, W. H. (2001). Growing up with parental alcohol abuse: Exposure to childhood abuse, neglect, and household dysfunction. *Child Abuse & Neglect, 25,* 1627-1640.

Dunn, M.G., Tarter, R.E., Mezzich, A.C., Vanyukov, M., Kirisci, L., & Kirillova, G. (2002). Origins and consequences of child neglect in substance abuse families. *Clinical Psychology Review, 22,* 1063-1090.

Easton, C.J., Swan, S., & Sinha, R. (2000). Prevalence of family violence in clients entering substance abuse treatment. *Journal of Substance Abuse Treatment, 18,* 23-28.

Ebrahim, S.H., Luman, E.T., Floyd, R.L., Murphy, C.C., Bennett, E.M., & Boyle, C.A. (1998). Alcohol consumption by pregnant women in the United States during 1988-1995. *Obstetrics & Gynecology, 92*(2), 187-191.

Edwards, M.E., & Steinglass, P. (1995). Family therapy outcomes for alcoholism. *Journal of Marital & Family Therapy, 21,* 475-509.

Eiden, R.D., Chavez, F., & Leonard, K.E. (1999). Parent-infant interactions among families with alcoholic fathers. *Development and Psychopathology, 11,* 745-762.

Eiden, R.D., & Leonard, K.E. (2000). Paternal alcoholism, parental psychopathology, and aggravation with infants. *Journal of Substance Abuse, 11*(1), 17-29.

Fals-Stewart, W., Birchler, G.R., & O'Farrell, T.J. (1999). Drug-abusing patients and their intimate partners: Dyadic adjustment, relationship stability, and substance use. *Journal of Abnormal Psychology, 108(1),* 11-23.

Famularo, R., Kinscherff, R., & Fenton, L. (1992). Parental substance abuse and the nature of child maltreatment. *Child Abuse & Neglect, 16,* 475-483.

Felitti, V. J., Anda, R.F., Nordenberg, D., Williamson, D. F., Spitz, A.M., Edwards, V., Koss, M.P., & Marks, J.S. (1998). Relationship of childhood abuse and household dysfunction to many of the leading causes of death in adults: The Adverse Childhood Experiences (ACE) Study. *American Journal of Preventive Medicine, 14*(4), 245-258.

Fiks, K.B., Johnson, H.L., & Rosen, T.S. (1985). Methadone-maintained mothers: 3-year follow-up of parental functioning. *The International Journal of the Addictions, 20,* 651-660.

Frank, D. A., Brown, J., Johnson, S., & Cabral H. (2002). Forgotten fathers: An exploratory study of mothers' report of drug and alcohol problems among fathers of urban newborns. *Neurotoxicology & Teratology, 24*(3), 339-347.

Froehlich, J.C., & Li, T.K., (1993). Opioid peptides. In M. Galante & H. Begleiter (Eds.), *Recent developments in alcoholism, Vol. 11: 10 years of progress.* (pp. 187-205). New York: NY: Plenum Press.

Gfroerer, J. (1987). Correlation between drug use by teenagers and drug use by older family members. *American Journal of Drug & Alcohol Abuse, 13,* 95-108.

Goodwin, D.W. (1995). Alcoholism and genetics: The sins of the fathers. *Archives of General Psychiatry 42,* 171-174.

Gorelick, D. A. (1993). Overview of pharmacologic treatment approaches for alcohol and other drug addiction: Intoxication, withdrawal, and relapse prevention. *Psychiatric Clinics of North America, 16*(1), 141-156.

Granfield, R., & Cloud, W. (2001). Social context and "natural recovery": The role of social capital in the resolution of drug-associated problems. *Substance Use & Misuse, 36*(11), 1543-1570.

Grant, B.F. (2000). Estimates of U.S. children exposed to alcohol abuse and dependence in the family. *American Journal of Public Health, 90,* 112-115.

Griffin, K.W., Botvin, G.J., Scheier, L.M., Diaz, T., & Miller, N.L. (2000). Parenting practices as predictors of substance use, delinquency, and aggression among urban minority youth: Moderating effects of family structure and gender. *Psychology of Addictive Behaviors, 14* (2), 174-184.

Gruber, K.J., Fleetwood, T.W., & Herring, M.W. (2001). In-home continuing care services for substance affected families: The Bridges Program. *Social Work, 46*(3), 267-277.

Gruber, K.J., & Fleetwood, T.W. (2004). In-home continuing care services for substance use affected families. *Substance Use & Misuse, 39*(9), 1381-1405.

Gutierres, S.E., Russo, N. F., & Urbanski, L. (1994). Sociocultural and psychological factors in American Indian drug use: Implications for treatment. *International Journal of the Addictions, 29,* 1761-1786.

Haber, J. (2000). Management of substance abuse and dependence problems in families. In M.A. Naegle & C.E. D'Avanzo (Eds.), *Addictions & substance abuse: Strategies for advanced practice nursing* (pp. 305-331). New Jersey: Prentice Hall.

Halford, W.K., & Osgarby, S.M. (1993). Alcohol abuse in clients presenting with marital problems. *Journal of Family Psychology, 6,* 245-254.

Hampton, R.L., Senatore, V., & Gullotta, T.P. (Eds.). (1998.) *Substance abuse, family violence, and child welfare: Bridging perspectives (Issues in children's and families' lives, Vol. 10).* Thousand Oaks, CA: Sage.

Hans, S. L. (2002). Studies of prenatal exposure to drugs: Focusing on parental care of children. *Neurotoxicology & Teratology, 24*(3), 329-337.

Hans, S. L., Bernstein, V. J., & Henson, L. G. (1999). The role of psychopathology in the parenting of drug-dependent women. *Development and Psychopathology, 11*(4), 957-977.

Harden, B.J. (1998). Building bridges for children: Addressing the consequences of exposure to drugs and to the child welfare system. In R.L. Hampton, V. Senatore, & T.P. Gullotta (Eds.), *Substance abuse, family violence, and child welfare: Bringing perspectives (Issues in children's and families' lives, Vol.10)* (pp. 18-61). Thousand Oaks, CA: Sage.

Hawkins, C. A. (1996). Pathogenic and protective relations in alcoholic families (II): Ritual invasion, shame, ACOA traits, and problem drinking in adult offspring. *Journal of Family Social Work, 1*(4), 51-63.

Hawkins, J.D., Catalano, R.F., & Miller, J.Y. (1992). Risk and protective factors for alcohol and other drug problems in adolescence and early adulthood: Implications for substance abuse prevention. *Psychological Bulletin, 112 (1),* 64-105.

Hawley, T.L., Halle, T.G., Drasin, R.E., & Thomas, N.G. (1995). Effects of the "crack epidemic" on the caregiving environment and the development of preschoolers. *American Journal of Orthopsychiatry, 65,* 364-379.

Hien, D., & Honeyman, T. (2000). A closer look at the drug abuse-maternal aggression link. *Journal of Interpersonal Violence, 15,* 503-522.

Hogue, A., Liddle, H. A., Becker, D., & Johnson-Leckrone, J. (2002). Family based prevention counseling for high risk young adolescents: Immediate outcomes. *Journal of Community Psychology, 30*(1), 1-22.

Hops, H., Tildesley, E., Lichestein, E., Ary, D., & Sherman, L. (1990). Parent-adolescent problem solving interactions and drug use. *American Journal of Drug and Alcohol Abuse, 16(3-4),* 239-258.

Hotaling, G.T., & Sugarman, D.B. (1986). An analysis of risk markers in husband to wife violence: The current state of knowledge. *Violence and Victims, 1,* 101-124.

Hurley, D.L. (1991). Women, alcohol, and incest: An analytic review. *Journal of Studies on Alcohol, 52,* 253-268.

Jang, K.L., Vernon, P.A, Livesley, W.J., Stein, M.B., & Wolf, H. (2001). Intra- and extra-familial influences on alcohol and drug misuse: A twin study of gene-environment correlation. *Addiction, 96,* 1307-1318.

Johnson, J. L., & Leff, M. (1999). Children of substance abusers: Overview of research findings. *Pediatrics, 103*(5), 1085-1099.

Johnson, K., Bryant, D.B., Collins, D.A., Noe, T.D., Strader, T.N., & Berbaum, M. (1998). Preventing and reducing alcohol and other drug use among high-risk youths by increasing family resilience. *Social Work, 43,* 297-308.

Johnson, G.M., Schoutz, F.C., & Locke, T.P. (1984). Relationships between adolescent drug use and parental drug behaviors. *Adolescence, 19,* 295-299.

Juliana, P., & Goodman, C. (1997). Children of substance abusing parents. In J.H. Lowinson, P. Ruiz, R.B. Millman, & J.G. Langrod (Eds.), *Substance abuse: A comprehensive textbook, 3rd Ed.* (pp.665-671). Baltimore: Lippincott, Williams, & Wilkins.

Kahler, C.W., McCrady, B.S., & Epstein, E.E. (2003). Sources of distress among women in treatment with their alcoholic partners. *Journal of Substance Abuse Treatment, 24,* 257-265.

Kantor, G. K., & Straus, M.A. (1989). Substance abuse as a precipitant of wife abuse victimizations. *American Journal of Drug and Alcohol Abuse, 15,* 173-189.

Kelley, M.L., & Fals-Stewart, W. (2002). Couple- versus individual-based therapy for alcohol and drug abuse: Effects on children's psychosocial functioning. *Journal of Consulting & Clinical Psychology, 70,* 417-427.

Kelley, S.J. (1992). Parenting stress and child maltreatment in drug-exposed children. *Child Abuse & Neglect, 16(3),* 317-328.

Knight, D.K, Hood, P.E., Logan, S.M., & Chatham, L.R. (1999). Residential treatment for women with dependent children: One agency's approach. *Journal of Psychoactive Drugs, 31,* 339-351.

Knight, D.K., & Simpson, D.D. (1996). Influences of family and friends on client progress during drug abuse treatment. *Journal of Substance Abuse, 8,* 417-429.

Kumpfer, K.L. (1987). Special populations: Etiology and prevention of vulnerability to chemical dependence in children of substance abusers. In B.S. Brown, & A.R. Mills (Eds.), *Youth at high risk for substance abuse* (pp. 1-71). Washington, DC: NIDA, DHHS.

Kumpfer, K.L., Alvarado, R., & Whiteside, H.O. (2003). Family-based interventions for substance use and misuse prevention. *Substance Use & Misuse, 38*(11-13), 1759-1787.

Lewchanin, S., & Sweeney, S. (1997). A developmental approach to the group treatment of adult children of alcoholics. *Alcoholism Treatment Quarterly, 15*(2), 51-62.

Li, C., Pentz, M.A., & Chou, C. (2002). Parental substance use as a modifier of adolescent substance use risk. *Addiction, 97,* 1537-1550.

Liddle, H.A., & Dakof, G.A. (1995). Efficacy of family therapy for drug abuse: Promising but not definitive. *Journal of Marital & Family Therapy, 21, 511-543.*

Lochman, J.E., & Steenhoven, A. (2002). Family-based approaches to substance abuse prevention. *The Journal of Primary Prevention, 23*(1), 49-114.

Luthar, S.S., Merikangas, K.R., & Rounsaville, B.J. (1993). Parental psychopathology and disorders in offspring: A study of relatives of drug abusers. *Journal of Nervous & Mental Disease, 181*(6), 351-357.

Lyter, L.L., & Lyter, S.C. (2003). Why some youth don't use alcohol: Protective factors and implications for parenting skills. *Social Work Practice in the Addictions 3*(2), 3-23.

Magura, S., & Laudet, A.B. (1996). Parental substance abuse and child maltreatment: review and implications for intervention. *Children and Youth Services Review, 18,* 193-220.

Margolis, R.D., & Zweben, J.E. (1998). *Treating patients with alcohol and other drug problems.* Washington, DC: American Psychological Association.

McCrady, B.S., & Epstein, E.E. (1995). Theoretical bases of family approaches to substance abuse treatment. In F. Rotger, D.S. Kekker, & J. Morganstern (Eds.), *Treating substance abuse: Theory and technique* (pp. 117-142). New York: Guilford Press

McCrady, B.S., Epstein, E.E., & Kahler, C.W. (1998). Families of alcoholics. In A. Bellack, & M. Hersen (Eds.), *Comprehensive clinical psychology: Vol 9. Applications in Diverse Populations* (pp. 199-218). New York: Elsevier.

McCubbin, H.I., McCubbin, M.A., Thompson, A.I., & Han, S. (1999). Contextualizing family risk factors for alcoholism and alcohol abuse. *Journal of Studies on Alcohol, Supplement No. 13,* 75-78.

McGillicuddy, N.B., Rychtarik, R.G., Duquette, J.A., & Morsheimer, E.T. (2001). Development of a skill training program for parents of substance-abusing adolescents. *Journal of Substance Abuse Treatment, 20,* 59-68.

McGue, M. (1993). From proteins to cognitions: The behavioral genetics of alcoholism. In R. Plomin & G.E. McClearn, (Eds). *Nature, nurture & psychology* (pp. 245-268). Washington, DC: American Psychological Association.

McIntyre, R.R (2004). Family treatment of substance abuse. In Straussner, S.L.A. (Ed.), *Clinical work with substance-abusing clients* (2nd ed.) (pp. 237-263). New York: Guilford Press.

McMahon, T.J., & Rounsaville, B.J. (2002). Substance abuse and fathering: Adding poppa to the research agenda. *Addiction 97,* 1109-1115.

McMahon, T.J., & Luthar, S.S. (1998). Bridging the gap for children as their parents enter substance abuse treatment. In R.L. Hampton, V. Senatore, & T.P. Gullotta (Eds.), *Substance abuse, family violence, and child welfare: Bridging Perspectives (Issues in Children's and Families' Lives, Vol.10)* (pp. 143-187). Thousand Oaks, CA: Sage.

McNichol, T., & Tash, C. (2001). Parental substance abuse and the development of children in foster care. *Child Welfare, 80*(2), 239-256.

Miller, B.A., Smyth, N.J., & Mudar, P.J. (1999). Mothers' alcohol and other drug problems and their punitiveness toward their children. *Journal of Studies on Alcohol, 60*(5), 632-642.

Moore, J., & Finkelstein, N. (2001). Parenting services for families affected by substance abuse. *Child Welfare, 80,* 221-238.

Moos, R.H., Finney, J.W., & Cronkite, R.C. (1990). *Alcoholism treatment: Context, process and outcome.* New York: Oxford University Press. RC 565 M67 1990.

Moss, H.B., Lynch, K.G., Hardie, T.L., & Baron, D.A. (2002). Family functioning and peer affiliation in children of fathers with antisocial personality disorder and substance dependence: Associations with problem behaviors. *American Journal of Psychiatry, 159,* 607-614.

Moss, H. B., Mezzich, A., Yao, J. K., Gavaler, J., & Martin, C.S. (1995). Aggressivity among sons of substance abusing fathers: Association with psychiatric disorders in the father and son, paternal personality, pubertal development, and socio-economic status. *American Journal of Drug and Alcohol Abuse, 21*(2), 195-208.

Mudar, P., Leonard, K.E., & Soltysinski, K. (2001). Discrepant substance use and marital functioning in newlywed couples. *Journal of Consulting & Clinical Psychology, 69(1),* 130-134.

Murray, J.B. (1989). Psychologists and children of alcoholic parents. *Psychological Reports, 64* (June, Part 1), 859-879.

National Institute on Drug Abuse, (1997) NIDA info facts. Retrieved June 27, 2003, from www.drugabuse.gov/Infofax/Infofaxindex.html

Needle, R., McCubbin, H., Wilson, M., Reineck, R., Lazar, A., Mederer, H. (1986). Interpersonal influences in adolescent drug use: The role of older siblings, parents, and peers. *International Journal of Addictions, 21,* 739-766.

Noll, R.B., Zucker, R.A., Fitzgerald, H.E., & Curtis, W.J. (1992). Cognitive and motoric functioning of sons of alcoholic fathers and controls: The early childhood years. *Developmental Psychology, 28*(4), 665-675.

O'Farrell, T. J. (Ed.) (1993). *Treating alcohol problems: Marital and family interventions.* New York: Guilford Press.

O'Farrell, T.J., & Fals-Stewart, W. (2000). Behavioral couples therapy for alcoholism and drug abuse. *Journal of Substance Abuse Treatment, 18,* 51-54.

Orford, J., Dalton, S., Hartney, E., Ferrins-Brown, M., Kerr, C., & Maslin, J. (2002). The close relatives of untreated heavy drinkers: Perspectives on heavy drinking and its effects. *Addiction Research and Theory, 10*(5), 439-463.

Orford, J., Natera, G., Velleman, R., Copello, A., Bowie, N., Bradbury, C., Davies, J., Mora, J., Nava, A., Rigby, K., & Tiburcio, M. (2001). Ways of coping and the health of relatives facing drug and alcohol problems in Mexico and England. *Addiction, 96*(5), 761-774.

Ossip-Klein, D. J., & Rychtarik, R.G. (1993). Behavioral contracts between alcoholics and family members: Improving aftercare participation and maintaining sobriety after inpatient alcoholism treatment. In T.J. O'Farrell (Ed.), *Treating alcohol problems: Marital and family interventions* (pp. 281–304). New York: Guilford Press.

Ragin, D. F., Pilotti, M., Madry, L., Sage, R.E., Bingham, L.E., & Primm, B.J. (2002). Intergenerational substance abuse and domestic violence as familial risk factors for lifetime attempted suicide among battered women. *Journal of Interpersonal Violence, 17*(10), 1027-1045.

Richardson, G.A., Ryan, C., Willford, J., Day, N.L., & Goldschmidt, L. (2002). Prenatal alcohol and marijuana exposure: Effects on neuropsychological outcomes at 10 years. *Neurotoxicology & Teratology, 24*(3), 309-320.

Rouse, B.A. (1998). *Substance Abuse and Mental Health Statistics Sourcebook.* Rockville, MD: Department of Health and Human Services, Substance Abuse and Mental health Services Administration, Office of Applied Studies

Sampson, P.D., Streissguth, A.P., Bookstein, F.L., Little, R.E., Clarren, S.K., Dehaene, P., Hanson, J.W., & Graham, J. M. (1997). Incidence of fetal alcohol syndrome and prevalence of alcohol-related neurodevelopmental disorder. *Teratology, 56*(5), 317-326.

Scharff, J.L., Broida, J.P., Conway, K., & Yue, A. (2004). The interaction of parental alcoholism, adaptation role, and familial dysfunction. *Addictive Behaviors, 29*(3), 575-581.

Semidei, J., Radel, L. F., & Nolan, C. (2001). Substance abuse and welfare: Clear linkages and promising responses. *Child Welfare, 80,* 109-128.

Sheridan, M.J. (1995). A proposed intergenerational model of substance abuse family functioning, and abuse/neglect. *Child Abuse & Neglect, 19, 519-530.*

Shuckit, M.A., & Smith, T.L. (2001). Correlates of unpredicted outcomes in sons of alcoholics and controls. *Journal of Studies on Alcohol, 62*(4), 477-485.

Stanton, M.D., & Shadish, W.R. (1997). Outcome, attrition, and family-couples treatment for drug abuse: A meta-analysis and review of the controlled, comparative studies. *Psychological Bulletin, 122,* 170-191.

Steinglass, P., Bennett, L.A., Wolin, S.J., & Reiss D. (1987). *The alcoholic family.* New York: Basic Books. HV5132.A44

Stevens-Smith, P. (1998). Maintaining behavior change: Relapse prevention strategies. In P. Stevens-Smith & R.L. Smith (Eds.), *Substance abuse counseling: Theory and practice.* New Jersey: Prentice Hall.

Stewart, M.A., & Brown, S.A. (1993). Family functioning following adolescent substance abuse treatment. *Journal of Substance Abuse, 5,* 327-339.

Straussner, S.L.A. (Ed.), (2004). *Clinical work with substance-abusing clients* (2nd ed.). New York: Guilford Press.

Stuart, G.L., Moore, T.M., Ramsey, S.E., & Kahler, C.W. (2003). Relationship aggression and substance use among women court-referred to domestic violence intervention programs. *Addictive Behaviors, 28,* 1603-1610.

Substance Abuse and Mental Health Services Administration, (2001). National Household Survey on Drug Abuse. Retrieved August 9, 2003, from htttp://www.samhsa.gov/centers/clearinghouse/clearinghouses.html

Suchman, N.E., & Luthar, S.S. (2000). Maternal addiction, child maladjustment, and social-demographic risks: Implications for parenting behaviors. *Addiction, 95,* 1417-1428.

Sullivan, W.P., Wolk, J.L., & Hartmann, D.J. (1992). Case management in alcohol and drug treatment: Improving client outcomes. *Families in Society, 73*(4), 195-202.

Thomas, E.J., & Ager, R. D. (1993). Unilateral family therapy with spouses of uncooperative alcohol abusers. In T.J. O'Farrell (Ed.), *Treating alcohol problems: Marital and family interventions* (pp. 3-33). New York: Guilford Press.

Thomas, C., & Corcoran, J. (2001). Empirically based marital and family interventions for alcohol abuse: A Review. *Research on Social Work Practice, 11*(5), 549-575.

Thompson, K.M., & Wilsnick, R.W. (1987). Parental influence on adolescent drinking: Modeling attitudes or conflict? *Youth and Society, 1987, 19,* 22-43.

Waldron, H.B. (1997). Adolescent substance abuse and family therapy outcome: A review of randomized trials. In T.H. Ollendick & R.J. Prinz (Eds.), *Advances in clinical child psychology (vol. 19)* (pp. 199-234). New York: Plenum Press.

Webb, J.A., Bray, J.H., Getz, J.G., & Adams, G.J. (2002). Gender, perceived parental monitoring, and behavioral adjustment: Influences on adolescent alcohol use. *American Journal of Orthopsychiatry, 72* (3), 392-400.

Weiss, R.D., Martinez-Raga, J., Griffin, M.L., Greenfield, S.F., & Hufford, C. (1997). Gender differences in cocaine dependent patients: A 6 month follow-up study. *Drug and Alcohol Dependence, 44,* 35-40.

West, M.O., & Prinz, R.J. (1987). Parental alcoholism and childhood psychopathology. *Psychological Bulletin, 102,* 204-218.

Wilsnack, S.C. (1996). Patterns and trends in women's drinking: Recent findings and some implications for prevention. *Women and Alcohol: Issues for Prevention Research. National Institute on Alcohol Abuse and Alcoholism. Research Monograph 32,* 19-63.

Wilsnack, S.C., & Wilsnack, R.W. (1993). Epidemiological research on women's drinking: recent progress and directions for the 1990s. In E.S.L.Gomberg & T.D. Nirenberg (Eds.), *Women and substance abuse* (pp. 62-99). Norwood, NJ: Ablex.

Wohlin, S.J., Bennett, L.A., Noonan, D.L., & Teitelbaum, M.A. (1980). Disrupted family rituals: A factor in the intergenerational transmission of alcoholism. *Journal of Studies on Alcohol, 41,* 199-214.

Wynne, R.D., McCrady, B.S., Kahler, C.W., Liddle, H.A., Palmer, R.B., Horberg, L.K., & Schlesinger, S.E. (1996). When addictions affect the family. In M. Harway (Ed.), *Treating the changing family* (pp. 293–317). New York: John Wiley & Sons.

Yamaguchi K., & Kandel, D.B. (1985). On the resolution of role incompatibility: A life event history analysis of family roles and marijuana use. *American Journal of Sociology, 9,* 1284-1325.

Zhang, L., Welte, J.W., & Wieczorek, W.F. (1999). The influence of parental drinking and closeness on adolescent drinking. *Journal of Studies on Alcohol, 60 (2),* 245-251.

Alcohol Problems, Marriage, and Treatment: Developing a Theoretical Timeline

Hilda Loughran

SUMMARY. While research findings over the past twenty years have consistently supported the efficacy of couples work with people experiencing alcohol related problems, in the field of practice in Ireland there is little evidence of the development of interventions based on a couples/marital perspective. This paper examines the place of marital work in the alcohol field through a review of the literature from 1950s to the present in order to discover the limitations in theory and research that might explain the reluctance of practitioners to adopt this method of intervention. *[Article copies available for a fee from The Haworth Document Delivery Service: 1-800-HAWORTH. E-mail address: <docdelivery@ haworthpress.com> Website: <http://www.HaworthPress.com> © 2006 by The Haworth Press, Inc. All rights reserved.]*

KEYWORDS. Alcohol problems, couples and marital treatment, research, outcomes

---

Hilda Loughran, PhD, CQSW, is affiliated with the Department of Social Policy and Social Work, University College Dublin, Dublin 4, Ireland (E-mail: hilda.loughran@ ucd.ie).

[Haworth co-indexing entry note]: "Alcohol Problems, Marriage, and Treatment: Developing a Theoretical Timeline." Loughran, Hilda. Co-published simultaneously in *Journal of Social Work Practice in the Addictions* (The Haworth Press, Inc.) Vol. 6, No. 1/2, 2006, pp. 31-48; and: *Impact of Substance Abuse on Children and Families: Research and Practice Implications* (ed: Shulamith Lala Ashenberg Straussner, and Christine Huff Fewell) The Haworth Press, Inc., 2006, pp. 31-48. Single or multiple copies of this article are available for a fee from The Haworth Document Delivery Service [1-800-HAWORTH, 9:00 a.m. - 5:00 p.m. (EST). E-mail address: docdelivery@ haworthpress.com].

Available online at http://www.haworthpress.com/web/JSWPA
doi:10.1300/J160v06n01_02

INTRODUCTION

This study resulted from the author's experience in developing treatment interventions with individuals with alcohol problems. Research studies indicate that work with a marital perspective would be beneficial to couples experiencing alcohol problems, yet there was limited evidence of such practice in the field in Ireland. The discrepancies between research findings and the translation of these findings into treatment services for problem drinkers inspired the current study, which aims at examining the past and current literature in order to identify the changing views and research activities on this topic over time.

METHOD

This article forms part of a larger qualitative study on alcohol problems and marriage from a treatment perspective (Loughran, 2002). It focuses on theory and practice pertaining to the development of ideas about the relationship between alcohol problems and marriage. This study examines the research on this topic during the time span from the 1950s to the present. The author interpreted the data through two key features: (1) the prevalence of a style or focus of research over a span of time, and (2) the implications for practice of the theoretical orientation identified. The chronological interpretation has been formulated into a series of stages that form a theoretical timeline analysis of research into alcohol problems and marriage, as illustrated in Figure 1. The time periods identified are indicative of research activities in those periods, rather than a definitive delineation.

FINDINGS AND DISCUSSION

The argument for considering the developments in the alcohol and marital intervention field will be discussed in relation to the proposed timeline. The phases identified by the author have been named: (1) curiosity about wives, (2) process phase, (3) family systems, (4) behavioral marital therapy, (5) Project MATCH, and (6) social networks. Each of these will be discussed in terms the data supporting their inclusion and their place on the timeline.

FIGURE 1. Alcohol Problems and Marriage: A Theoretical Timeline

1950s: Curiosity About Wives Phase	Curiosity about wives of alcoholics. Lack of information about spouses of alcoholics led to a range of exploratory research looking at the role of spouses in the addiction process and the personalities of women married to "alcoholics."
1960s: Process-Focused Phase	Concern about the nature of marital interaction and its connection to alcoholism. Still struggling with theoretical restrictions imposed by disease perspectives. Work being conducted at more theoretical than research level looking at issues such as communication patterns.
1970s: Family Systems Phase	Sustained interest in process, but now supported by developing framework of systems theory. Conjoint work legitimized by the establishment of family systems theory as an alternative conceptual framework. Studies into the importance of including spouses within a family therapy framework. This phase represented an attempt to integrate emerging systemic theories into work with couples and families dealing with alcoholism.
1980s: Treatment-focused Phase or Behavioral Marital Therapy (BMT Phase)	Failure of systems ideas to penetrate clinical arena in alcohol research or treatment weakened family approaches in terms of research methodology. Translation of marital concerns into behavioral approaches. Effectiveness of treatment the central concern. Behavioral Marital Therapy dominating research and "proving" its superiority as a treatment approach. Studies focused on treatment outcome and quantitative research.
1990s: Project MATCH and Post Project MATCH Phase	Continuance of BMT dominance until mid-1990s. Post Project MATCH generating questions about the evidence that behavioral approaches offered. Re-emerging uncertainty coincided with social constructionist thinking being applied to alcohol field.
2000 to date: Social Networks Phase	Influenced by project MATCH and the Community Reinforcement Movement, interest in spouses appears to be subsumed under the umbrella term of social network or social supports. This represents an expansion of interest and reflects the public health debate on alcohol problems in the population at large. It also suggests a recognition of the connection between the personal experience of alcohol problems and the social context within which problem drinking develops and is maintained.

Curiosity About Wives Phase (1950s)

When alcoholism is conceptualized within an "individual disease" framework, then the inclusion of the spouse may be unnecessary. The rationale for engaging in research into alcoholism and the inclusion of spouses is dependent on developing theories of the role of spouses in the addiction equation. The debate about wives of alcoholics was fueled by a report from Whelan in 1953, which attempted to distinguish a variety of spousal "types." The four types identified–the sufferer, the controller, the waverer, and the punisher–gained a significant place in addiction folklore.

Whelan's (1953) position was that although alcoholism is an illness it is not a clinical entity like, for example, typhoid fever; that it will assume different forms in different individuals and that therefore there is no uniform treatment procedure. She proposed the view that "the wife of an alcoholic is not simply the object of mistreatment in a situation which she has no part in creating, her personality was just as responsible for the making of this marriage as her husband was, and in the sordid sequence of marital misery which follows she is not an innocent bystander" (p. 634). This poses challenges to the conceptualization of the addiction dynamic of the alcoholic as having a disease. The diversity promoted by Whelan (1953) was superseded by a more homogeneous view of the problem of alcoholism.

Joan Jackson (1954) further explored the role wives might play in the addiction process. Jackson traced the adjustment by wives reported having to their husbands' alcoholism. She suggested that wives may accommodate or enable their husbands' alcoholism because of the manner in which they learn to live with the crises caused by their drinking. Jackson detailed seven stages in the adjustment to alcoholism. These were (1) attempts to deny the problem, (2) attempts to eliminate the problem, (3) disorganization, (4) attempts to reorganize in spite of the problems, (5) efforts to escape the problems, (6) reorganization of part of the family, and, finally, (7) recovery and reorganization of all the family.

Early research studies, such as those by Gliedman, Rosenthal, Frank, and Nash (1956) and MacDonald (1958), indicated that the inclusion of spouses in some forms of treatment might be beneficial. These studies had limited methodological bases and did not employ control groups or use standardized measures to evaluate success. Nonetheless, the indication that the spouse might benefit from treatment set the ground for further investigation. MacDonald (1958) identified the possibility that "neurotic" wives might complement the needs of alcoholic husbands. If this proved to be the case, then both spouses would need to be in treatment.

These studies, which considered the part the spouse played in the addiction, raised questions about the interpersonal relationship between spouses and their alcoholic partners. The question of whether there is any benefit to inclusion of spouses in treatment highlights a complex research issue. It becomes necessary to ask whether spousal involvement in treatment incorporates an attempt to change behavior on the part of both spouse and alcoholic, as Whelan (1953) suggested, or whether evidence of abstinence, which represents change in the alcoholic's behavior only, can be considered a sufficient gauge?

While this phase did contribute to a discussion about the role of the spouse in addiction, it did not offer a theoretical explanation about the part a spouse might play in the development of the addiction. The dominant thinking of the time continued to focus on a disease causation model. From a treatment perspective the most influential development was to draw attention to the needs of spouses. There was recognition that any treatment intervention should at least acknowledge that spouses were affected by the problem drinking. This recognition lead to a shift in interest to looking at the mechanisms within a marriage that may facilitate or hinder communication about the drinking.

Process-Focused Phase (1960s)

While research was still influenced by the earlier psychopathology approach to spouses, one of the most striking features of this phase was the attempt to look beyond the effects of alcohol to the role of communication between the spouses and to compare this with communication in non-alcoholic marriages. Hanson, Sands, and Sheldon (1968) investigated whether communication problems preceded or were directly related to drinking problems. They suggested that "the alcoholic is some-what of a mystery to his spouse" (p. 546). They concluded that communication was a problem within these marriages, but felt further study would be required to answer questions of causation.

Drewery and Rae (1969) also attempted to study communication patterns between spouses. They concluded that alcoholic couples engaged in conflict about dependence and independence within the marriage. This finding continued to influence thinking on interaction between spouses. Possibly, this was the forerunner to the view of the overly dependent spouse, who was later conceptualized as being a codependent (Brown 1990; Humes, 1989). Research efforts in this phase appear to have been hampered by the fact that theory had not yet developed a framework to encapsulate the complexity of the interactions between spouses. While research was directed at increasing understanding of the part of spouses in the process, there was no attempt made to challenge the underlying belief that alcoholism was a disease. There is little evidence of substantial research during this phase. The work of Drewery and Rae (1969) was influenced by the emerging systems movement and represents the start of the shift into the next phase.

Family Systems Phase (1970s)

In the seventies, interest in systems thinking and addiction emerges in the literature. The early work on mixed alcoholic and non-alcoholic marital couples groups by Cadogan (1973) attempted to apply quantitative methodology to the subject of couples' treatment in a marital group setting. Cadogan (1973) established a control group and a treatment group and evaluated the effect of treatment on abstinence and the effect of treatment on dealing with alcohol-related problems. Cadogan concluded that a key issue in predicting abstinence was the level of trust and acceptance the non-drinking spouse had in his/her drinking partner prior to starting treatment. The number of prior episodes of treatment was clearly linked to the level of trust and acceptance. Previous failure in treatment had a negative impact on trust and acceptance. The nature of this trust and acceptance, however, was not explored, nor was the question of what factors enabled the spouses to maintain belief in their partners in spite of years of alcohol-related difficulties. Indeed, what the previous treatment experience contributed to the decline in the spouse's ability to trust her partner was not explored at all.

This phase incorporated a growing interest in understanding the similarities and differences between "alcoholic" and "normal" marriages. Drewery and Rae (1969) and Gorad (1972) all contributed to this alcoholic versus "non-alcoholic" debate. The evidence of these studies overturned a commonly held view, dating from Whelan (1953), that wives dominated alcoholic husbands. The validity of the Drewery and Rae (1969) finding, however, could be called into question when the methodology of the research is considered. Given that the nature of the measurement tool was a card game designed around the goal of making money, the social context for participants was significant. Important variables, such as educational and income levels of the subjects, were not controlled for. The "alcoholic couples" were on average less educated, and earned only half or less than half the income of the "normal couples." Issues related to money matters, therefore, may have had a totally different meaning to the two sets of couples, above and beyond any issue to do with alcohol use. The task of establishing that "alcoholic couples" are qualitatively different than "non-alcoholic couples" has been a very difficult one. To date, the information remains inconclusive.

By 1975, Orford (1975) summarized the situation when he wrote "two models have dominated the literature on 'alcoholism' and marriage. One emphasizes the 'psychopathology' of the wives of alcoholics, while the second takes the view that the behavior of wives may be understood as the reactions of 'normal' women to the crisis or stress occasioned by their husband's excessive drinking" (p. 1254). The future direction of research was clearly influenced by these dominant models.

Studies that attempted to recreate the circumstances of intoxication were popular in the 1970s and some innovative research methods were developed in this phase, such as the use of experimental intoxication research (Steinglass, Davis, & Berenson, 1977). Although this method did provide unique insights into the world of alcohol and marital communication, the ethical questions about allowing, indeed encouraging, intoxication for research purposes have terminated this type of study methodology. Some of the most controversial findings in the addiction field can be attributed to these types of study.

In one of the well-known studies of this type, Steinglass, Davis, and Berenson (1977) studied conjointly hospitalized couples. Their decision to include "experimentally induced intoxication" is seen as a reason why there were difficulties getting volunteers for the study. They observed "non random and in this sense even more highly patterned behavior in intoxication compared with sobriety. There was little evidence of anticipated impulsive, explosive and unanticipated behaviour" (p. 12). This was interpreted as further evidence of the stability offered by intoxication within the marriage.

Hersen, Miller, and Eisler (1973) observed that "wives looked more at their husbands during interactions related to the husband's drinking problems than during interaction unrelated to drinking. In contrast, the duration of looking by husbands was slightly longer during non-alcohol-related interactions" (p. 518). These findings were interpreted as spousal reinforcement of the alcohol-related interactions.

Paolino and McCrady (1977) developed a theoretical framework for understanding the role of alcoholism in a marriage. They suggested that the symptom of alcoholism in the family may have a useful function in keeping families together and creating or maintaining stability within the family system. They hypothesized that, theoretically, alcoholics may be signaling distress in the family, or that they may be stepping back from responsibility to avoid conflict. There was an indication that some families might not survive without the symptom, but at that time the possibility that alcoholism was transmitted through intergenerational family communication patterns had not yet been researched. Work on this aspect of family dynamics would continue into the 1980s.

Steinglass (1980, 1981) and his colleagues (Steinglass, Tisenko, and Reiss 1985; Steinglass et al., 1987) studied the lives of families living with alcoholism to try to develop theoretical insights that could be the foundation of treatment interventions. They were particularly interested in the resilience of children living with alcoholism. Understanding how some children emerge intact from alcoholic families could be used to create a prevention approach to working with families. These studies succeeded in keeping the interest in family-based treatment models alive, but they continued to have little influence on ideas about the etiology of alcoholism or the development of alternatives to the medical model treatment approach.

Work being conducted by Hunt and Azrin (1973) at this time was looking at family from the broader context of social networks. Their ideas conceived in the 1970s would re-emerge in the new millennium. However by the 1980s other avenues of investigation took prominence. These related to the emergence of the influential behavioral school, which is supported by a strong and prolific research base.

Behavioral Marital Therapy (BMT) Phase (1980s)

McCrady (1982, 1989) and McCrady and colleagues (McCrady & Hay 1987; McCrady, Noel, Abrams, Stout, Neban, & Hay, 1986; and McCrady, Stout, Noel, Abrams, & Fisher-Nelson, 1991) pursued research of Behavioral Marital Therapy (BMT). Others, such as O'Farrell and Cutter (1984), developed a Behavioral Marital Therapy Couples Group (BMT). O'Farrell and Cutter (1984) found that couples who complete BMT couples group reported higher levels of relationship satisfaction, demonstrated greater marital stability, and displayed more positive communication skills while discussing marital issues.

Several variations of BMT became major areas of research. Studies compared behavioral therapies of different intensity and duration, compared control groups with those receiving other forms of therapy, and looked at combinations of inpatient and outpatient groups (Bowers & Al Redha, 1990; Maisto, McKay, & O'Farrell, 1997; McCrady, 1989; 1991; McCrady et al., 1986; McNabb, Der Karabetian, & Rhoads, 1989; O'Farrell et al., 1993; O'Farrell, Choquette, & Cutter, 1998; O'Farrell & Cutter, 1984; O'Farrell, Cutter, & Floyd, 1985). All supported the view that including the spouse was beneficial and reported the superiority of BMT as a treatment approach.

The position of behavioral treatment was further supported in several reviews of research that were conducted through the late-eighties and early-nineties. Holder, Longabaugh, Miller, and Rubonis (1991) found that behavioral marital treatment was cost-effective compared to other forms of treatments. Miller and Hester (1980) had identified and reviewed 579 studies related to alcoholism treatment. One of the short-comings of this review, as identified by Miller and Hester in 1995, was the lack of weighting which would have differentiated between the methodological qualities of the research conducted. Redressing this limitation, Miller and Hester (1995) defined 219 studies as being suitable for inclusion. The weighting was specifically related to the demands of quantitative research methods. This emphasis on positivistic rigor echoed the earlier problems identified with regard to systems-based marital treatments. Behavioral marital treatment was well represented in this review and performed favorably overall. The challenge of this type of review, however, is to represent the diversity of research methods across the quantitative/qualitative divide. Miller and Hester (1995) did not address this issue. As a result, the contribution of BMT may have been overvalued over other less-researched treatments or treatments that were inaccessible to mainstream quantitative methods, an issue raised as early as 1982 by McCrady.

Despite the evidence emerging from the behavioral studies that BMT was effective, there was little evidence of a reorientation of treatment alternatives. The developments, both in terms of new understandings of the etiology of addiction and related treatment potentials, were slow to find a foothold within a traditional alcoholism treatment industry. Whatever the retrospective interpretation, the future domination of behavioral treatment and research would be challenged by the findings of a major research study, Project MATCH (Matching Alcoholism Treatment to Client Heterogeneity), funded by the National Institute on Alcohol Abuse and Alcoholism, which published its findings in the mid-1990s.

Project MATCH and Post Project MATCH Phase (1990s)

During the late 1980s, both Marlatt (1988) and Miller (1989) addressed the issue of matching clients to specific interventions. The concept of matching revolves around two central points; firstly, the recognition that individuals have different experiences of addiction and therefore have different needs, and, secondly, that different interventions can be offered to clients. As interest in matching grew, Mattson and Allan (1991) reviewed the research on matching patients to treatment. They reported that although the concept of matching posed problems in terms of developing research protocol, it none-the-less "offers considerable promise to improve the treatment of alcoholism" (p. 46). Project MATCH was designed to test this matching hypothesis and the question of what criteria could be employed to select or match clients with an intervention was addressed in this research (Project MATCH Research Group, 1993).

Project MATCH has generated many reports and much debate in the alcohol treatment field (Addiction (Special Edition), 1999; Longabaugh & Wirtz, 2001; Project MATCH Research Group, 1998). This is indicative of its importance in addiction discourse. It has, therefore, been incorporated into this study even though no couple interventions were included in the research (in spite of the fact that 36% of the outpatient sample and 34% of the aftercare sample in the study were registered as being part of a couple). From a marital alcohol-research perspective, the absence of a dedicated marital intervention is disheartening. The prolific research in the Behavioral Marital Therapy field did not ensure a place for a couples approach in this multi-million dollar study (a reported $26 million, according to Drummond, 1999). In fact, all three models used in the study (Motivational Enhancement Therapy, Cognitive Behavioral Therapy, and Twelve Step Facilitation Therapy) were primarily directed at individual interventions. The absence of both group therapy and couples therapy suggest that the designers of the project were more focused on content material that could be put into manuals than on process (the interpersonal interactions related to the ways in which the content would be delivered). On reviewing the project, it appears that while the goal was to explore heterogeneity and matching, the final manualized models were not reflective of the variety of treatment interventions utilized in the field.

An important finding from this research was the recognition that there were multiple factors to be considered in defining treatment procedures and in assessing success. Epstein, McCrady, Miller, and Steinberg (1994) commented that "as the literature on heterogeneity of the alcoholic population grows, assessment and diagnostic information may become important in the treatment service area" (p. 259). There developed a growing school of thought that perhaps it was necessary to be more flexible about treatment possibilities.

The results of this major project were surprising in that there was little difference in outcomes among the three intervention approaches used. One critic (Glasser, 1999) commented, "A possible whimsical simile suggests itself: Project MATCH as the Titanic of treatment outcome studies. Like Project MATCH, the great ship was large, the largest man-made object to that point in history. It was complex, it generated enormous enthusiasm; and it sank like a stone on its maiden voyage with great loss of life" (p. 34).

In the present study, Project MATCH and Post Project MATCH have been identified as a marker in the summary timeline developed by the author. Its significance is that it marks the failure of couples' intervention research to establish itself as a major player in alcoholism research. It also confirms that hitherto under-researched approaches were competitive with the researched approaches. The unexpected and disappointing results of Project MATCH raised questions about methodological issues. Miller (2002) reflected on the possibility that treatment manuals designed to satisfy the rigors of research may detract from the specific qualities of the methods being evaluated. Project MATCH (Project MATCH Research Group 1997) reviewed both abstinence and number of drink-free days in its analysis. This reveals an underlying assumption that goals other than total abstinence have a place in alcohol treatment and research. And finally, from the extensive attempts to learn from the experience, the issue of social networks emerged as a topic deserving future research. While it is still premature to predict the next phase, this study proposes that the resurgence of interest in social networks will leave its mark on the timeline of research about alcohol problems.

Social Networks Phase (2000 to date)

Hester and Miller (1989) warned of the danger that conflicting research results might lead to a belief that nothing works or that one approach is just as valid as all others. They dismiss these beliefs as myths. They did, however, accept that there is some evidence that alcoholics may achieve sobriety without the aid of treatment. This is sometimes referred to as spontaneous recovery. This idea has been expanded to include consideration of remission without treatment (Bischof, Rumpe, Hapke, Meyer, & John, 2002). It is worth noting Cunningham's report (1999) on the effectiveness of treatments. He applied a variety of levels of alcohol-related problems as defining criteria for inclusion as problem drinking. He also regarded improvement to include both abstinence and moderate drinking. Cunningham (1999) commented that "while the present analysis closely replicates earlier findings [referring to 78% untreated recoveries in Sobell, Cunningham, and Sobell, 1996], it also demonstrates the variability that can be obtained in estimates of untreated recoveries by changing the criteria for defining a prior alcohol problem" (p. 465).

In the face of this uncertainty, new issues have attracted the attention of researchers in the field. One of the contributions of Project MATCH was to draw attention to the question of social networks. The Project MATCH finding that network support for drinking was one of the factors that was prognostic of drinking outcomes rekindled interest in the issue. This was not a new issue in the field of alcohol research: Barber and Crisp (1995b) found that the most supportive individual in the drinker's social network had an important influence on successful outcome. Zywiak, Longabaugh, and Wirtz (2002) note that "two decades ago, investigators sought to disentangle the conceptual ambiguity of social support in alcohol treatment research" (p. 114). They clarify the distinction between support for the patient regarding attempts to remain abstinent and support for the patient's general well-being.

The importance of social networks in impacting on drinking behavior is central to the community reinforcement approach (Hunt & Azrin, 1973). The community reinforcement approach incorporates family and spousal relationships as part of the much broader definition of network. Hunt and Azrin's approach to networks was not incorporated into the systemic thinking of the 1970s, but remained part of a discussion which emanated more from a health promotion than a family therapy perspective. Miller, Meyers, and Tonigan (1999) have turned their attention to community reinforcement treatment. The inclusion of the broader social environment is evidenced by these developments. One might speculate that the advances in research in the wider addiction arena have influenced this expansion beyond the individual to incorporate more social dimensions.

Sobell, Sobell, and Leo (2000) studied the issue of social support networks in marital relationships. In their study they recruited drinkers and their spouses into brief outpatient treatment conditions, those in the natural support group (NS), and those assigned to a directed support group (DS). The NS condition were not given any explicit instruction to be supportive of their partner's changes, while the DS condition was to have the spouse become a continuing agent of treatment with an emphasis on support in drinker's aftercare. Both groups were reported to have made and maintained improvement at one year follow up, but no difference was found between the groups. This study focused attention on the role of the spouse in the social network debate. The continued emphasis on the spouse as a supporter and motivator fails to address the more systemic nature of the marital relationship, although it has put marital relations back on the agenda.

In the United States the interest in social support networks resulted in the development of Community Reinforcement and Family Treatment (CRAFT) (Miller, Meyers, & Hiller-Sturmhofel (1999). In the United

Kingdom the social network and community reinforcement elements have been developed into a treatment entitled Social Behavior and Network Therapy (SBNT). The principles of the treatment, resulting from initial studies, were presented by Copello et al. (2002). The approach identifies family members and concerned others as central to treatment. The SBNT movement, along with other studies mentioned, supports the suggestion that interest in understanding and developing the social network construct can justifiably be seen as the current phase in alcohol studies. The prospect that this phase heralds a new and invigorating era in alcohol and marital treatment and research is, however, threatened by a number of concerns. The emphasis on social networks appears to have recruited more interest in pharmaceutical responses to alcohol problems (O'Farrell, Allen, & Litten, 1995), including a new major project in the USA–Project COMBINE (Miller, 1999), and the emphasis relating to spouses continues to be focused mainly on engagement and retention of the alcoholic in treatment.

The Social Network Phase, as identified in this research, is consistent with developments in the public health debate on alcohol problems as they affect the population at large. The Social Network approach mirrors elements of the community reinforcement model. These have been adopted in the public policy approach to tackling levels of alcohol use that would not be defined as dependent use, but which nonetheless are the cause of serious problems for drinkers and society. These network/community approaches could be seen as part of the broader systems approach to alcohol problems since systems ideas support the inclusion of wider family and social factors in the consideration of problem development. However, in the context of the research reviewed in this study, these social network and community reinforcement approaches are situated predominantly within the cognitive behavioral school of thought. Within this exploration of networks, the marital domain should assert its significance. However, it does appear that larger systems, such as the alcohol industry itself, are more likely to be the target of change in this approach.

It is, of course, possible that the BMT Phase identified as being dominant in the 1990s is only in recession. The impact of the abundance of research in the behavioral field should not be under-estimated. It continues to be cited by Copello et al. (2002) as a treatment that is "among those with greatest evidence of positive treatment outcome" (p. 346), and by Miller and Wilbourne (2002) who state that "among psychosocial treatments, strongest evidence of efficacy was found for brief interventions, social skills training, the community reinforcement approach, behavior contracting, behavioral marital therapy and case management" (p. 265).

CONCLUSION

In 1999, Leonard and Rothbard revisited the topic of alcohol problems and marriage. Their findings support the need to inquire further into the nature of the relationship between marriage and the development and/or maintenance of alcohol problems. They also encourage family and marital clinicians to develop treatment models consistent with the concepts and principles of family systems theory, and, within those marital interventions, to deal with alcohol problems. These developments, overall, provide a rationale for further investigating the connection between alcohol problems and interpersonal relationships, specifically marital relations. They justify renewed interest in alcohol use as part of a life transition and developmental phase.

The theoretical timeline offered here provides a resource to those interested in the place of couples' interventions in the treatment of alcohol problems. It acknowledges key contributions to the field and identifies some of the issues that may be inhibiting progress in the development of related treatment interventions.

REFERENCES

Barber, J., & Crisp, B. (1995). The pressures to change approach to working with the partners of heavy drinkers. *Addiction*, 90: 269-276.

Bischof, G., Rumpe, H., Hapke, U., Meyer, C., & John, U. (2002). Remission from alcohol dependence without help: How restrictive should our definition of treatment be? *Journal of Studies on Alcohol*, 63: 229-236.

Bowers, T., & Al-Redha, M. (1990) A comparison of outcome with group/marital and standard/individual therapies with alcoholics. *Journal of Studies on Alcohol*, 51:4: 301-309.

Brown, L.S. (1990). What's addiction got to do with it: A feminist critque of co-dependency. *Psychology of Women*, Newsletter Division 35, American Psychological Association 17: Winter 1-4.

Cadogan, D. (1973). Marital group therapy in the treatment of alcoholism. *Quarterly Journal of Studies on Alcohol*, 34: 1187-1194.

Copello, A., Orford, J., Hodgson, R., Tober, G., & Barrett, C. (2002). Social behavior and network therapy: Basic principles and early experiences. *Addictive Behaviors*, 27: 345-366.

Cunningham, J. (1999). Resolving alcohol-related problems with and without treatment: The effects of different problem criteria. *Journal of Studies on Alcohol*, 60: 463-466.

Donovan, M., & Marlatt, A. (Eds.) (1988). *Assessment of Addictive Behaviours*, New York, Guilford Press.

Drewery, J., & Rae, J. (1969). A group comparison of alcoholic and non alcoholic marriages using the interpersonal perception technique. *British Journal of Psychiatry*, 115: 287-300.

Drummond, D. (1999). Treatment research in the wake of Project MATCH. *Addiction*, 94: 39-42.

Epstein, E., McCrady, B., Miller, K., & Steinberg, M. (1994). Attrition from conjoint alcoholism treatment: Do dropouts differ from completers? *Journal of Substance Abuse*, 6: 249-265.

Glaser, F. (1999). The unsinkable Project MATCH. *Addiction*, 94: 34-36.

Gliedman, L., Rosenthal, D., Frank, J., & Nash, H. (1956). Group therapy of alcoholics with concurrent meetings with their wives. *Quarterly Journal of Studies on Alcohol*, 17: 655-670.

Gorad, S. (1972). Communication styles and interactions of alcoholics and their wives. *Family Process*, 10 (4): 651-668.

Hanson, P., Sands, P., & Sheldon, R. (1968). Patterns of communication in alcoholic marital couples. *Psychiatry Quarterly*, 42:538-547.

Heather, N. (1996). The public health and brief interventions for excessive alcohol consumption: The British experience. *Addictive Behaviors*, 21 (6) 857-868.

Hersen, M., Miller, P., & Eisler, R. (1973). Interactions between alcoholics and their wives; a descriptive analysis of verbal and nonverbal behavior, *Quarterly Journal of Studies on Alcohol*, 34: 516-520.

Hester, R., & Miller, W. (Eds.) (1989). *Handbook of Alcoholism Treatment Approaches, Effective Alternatives*. Boston: Pergamon.

Hester, R., & Miller, W. (Eds.) (1995). *Handbook of Alcoholism Treatment Approaches, Effective Alternatives* (2nd ed.), Boston: Allyn and Bacon.

Holder, H., Longabaugh, R., Miller, W., & Rubonis, A. (1991) The cost effectiveness of treatment for alcoholism: A first approximation. *Journal of Studies on Alcohol*, 52:517-540.

Humes, A. (1989). The culture of co-dependency. *7 Days*, 21:26.

Hunt, G., & Azrin, N. (1973). A community reinforcement approach to alcoholism. *Behavior Research and Therapy*, 11:91-104.

Jackson, J. (1954). The adjustment of the family to the crisis of alcoholism. *Quarterly Journal of Studies on Alcohol*, 15: 562-586.

Leonard, K., & Rothbard, J. (1999). Alcohol and Marriage Effect. *Journal of Studies on Alcohol Supplement*, 13:139-146.

Longabaugh, R., Wirtz, P., Zweben, A., & Stout, R. (2001). Network support for drinking, in Longabaugh, R. and Wirtz, P. (Eds.), *Project MATCH Hypothesis: Results and causal chain analysis*, Rockville, MD: National Institute on Alcohol Abuse and Alcoholism, Project MATCH Monograph Series, Volume 8: 260-275.

Loughran, H. (2002). *A Study of Alcohol Problems and Marriage from a Treatment Perspective*, Unpublished PhD thesis, University College Dublin, Ireland.

MacDonald, D. (1956). Mental disorders in wives of alcoholics. *Quarterly Journal of Studies on Alcohol*, 17 (2): 282-287.

MacDonald, D. (1958). Group psychotherapy with wives of alcoholics. *Quarterly Journal of Studies on Alcohol*, 19 (1): 125-132.

Maisto, S., McKay, J., & O'Farrell, T. (1997). Twelve-month abstinence from alcohol and long-term drinking and marital outcomes in men with severe alcohol problems. *Journal of Studies on Alcohol*, 59: 591-598.

Marlatt, A. (1988). Matching clients to treatment: Treatment models and stages of change. In Donovan, M. and Marlatt, A. (Eds.). *Assessment of Addictive Behaviors*, (pp. 474-483). New York: Guilford Press.

Mattson, M., & Allen, J. (1991). Research on matching alcoholic patients to treatments: Findings, issues, and implications. *Journal of Addictive Diseases*, 11 (2) 33-49.

McCrady, B. (1982). Marital dysfunction: Alcoholism and marriage. In Pattison, E. and Kaufman, E. (Ed.). *Encyclopaedic Handbook of Alcoholism*, (pp. 673-681). New York: Gardner Press.

McCrady, B. (1989). Extending relapse prevention models to couples. *Addictive Behaviors*, 14: 69-74.

McCrady, B. (1991). Promising but underutilized treatment approaches. *Alcohol Health and Research World*, 15: 215-218.

McCrady, B., & Hay, W. (1987). Coping with problem drinking in the family. In Orford, J. (Eds.). *Coping with Disorder in the Family*, (pp. 86-116). Beckenham: Croom Helm.

McCrady, B., Moreau, J., Paolino, T., & Longabaugh, R. (1982). Joint hospitalization and couples therapy for alcoholism: A four-year follow-up. *Journal of Studies on Alcohol*, 43 (11): 1244-1249.

McCrady, B., Noel, N., Abrams, D., Stout, R., Neban, H., & Hay, W. (1986). Comparative effectiveness of three types of spouse involvement in outpatient behavioural alcoholism treatment. *Journal of Studies on Alcohol*, 47 (6) 459-467.

McCrady, B., Paolino, T., Longabaugh, R., & Rossi, J. (1979). Effects of joint hospital admission and couples treatment for hospitalized alcoholics: A pilot study. *Addictive Behaviors*, 4: 155-165.

McCrady, B., Stout, R., Noel, N., Abrams, D., & Fisher-Nelson, H. (1991). Effectiveness of three types of spouse involved alcohol treatment: Outcomes 18 months after treatment. *British Journal of Addiction*, 86: 1415-1424.

McNabb, J., Der-Karabetian, A., & Rhoads, J. (1989). Family involvement and outcome in treatment of alcoholism. *Psychological Reports*, 65: 1327-1330.

Miller, W. (1989). Matching individuals with interventions. In Hester, R. & Miller, W. (Eds.). *Handbook of Alcoholism Treatment Approaches* (pp. 261-271). *Effective Alternatives*, New York: Pergamon Press.

Miller, W. (2002). MINT Conference, Hawaii.

Miller, W., & Heather, N. (Eds) (1998). *Treating addictive behaviors* (2nd ed). New York: Plenum Press.

Miller, W., & Hester, R. (1980). Treating problem drinkers: Modern approaches. In Miller, W. (Eds.). *The Addictive Behaviors: Treatment of Alcoholism, Drug Abuse, Smoking, and Obesity* (11-141). Oxford: Pergamon Press.

Miller, W., & Hester, R. (1995). The effectiveness of alcoholism treatment methods: What research reveals. In Miller, W. and Heather, N. (Eds.). *Treating Addictive Behaviors: Processes of Change* (2nd ed.) (pp. 121-174). New York: Plenum Press.

Miller, W., & Wilbourne, P. (2002). Mesa Grande: A methodological analysis of clinical trials of treatments for alcohol use disorders. *Addiction*, 97:265-277.

Miller, W., Meyers, R., & Hiller-Sturmhofel, S. (1999). The community-reinforcement approach. *Alcohol Research and Health*, 23 (2): 116-121.

Miller, W., Meyers, R., & Tonigan, J. (1999). Engaging the unmotivated in treatment for alcohol problems: A comparison of three strategies for intervention through family members. *Journal of Consulting & Clinical Psychology*, 67(5): 688-697.

O'Farrell, T. (1993). A behavioral marital therapy couples group program for alcoholics and their spouses. In O'Farrell, T. (Ed.). *Treating Alcohol Problems: Marital and Family Interventions*, (pp.170-209). New York: Guilford Press.

O'Farrell, T., Qllen, J., & Litten, R. (1995). Disulfiram (Antabuse) contracts in treatment of alcoholism. In NIDA, Integrating Behaviorial Therapies with Medication in the Treatment of Drug Dependence, NIDA, Monograph No. 15; 65-91.

O'Farrell, T., Choquette, K., & Cutter, H. (1998). Couples relapse prevention sessions after behavioral marital therapy for male alcoholics: Outcomes during the three years after starting treatment. *Journal of Study on Alcohol*, 59:357-370.

O'Farrell, T., Choquette, K., Cutter, H., Brown, E., & McCourt, W. (1993). Behavioral marital therapy with and without additional couples relapse prevention sessions for alcoholics and their wives. *Journal of Studies in Alcohol*, 54: 652-666.

O'Farrell, T., Cutter, H., & Floyd, F. (1985). Evaluating behavioral marital therapy for male alcoholics: Effects on marital adjustment and communication from before and after treatment. *Behavior Therapy*, 16, 147-167.

O'Farrell, T., Cutter, H., Choquette, K., Floyd, F., & Bayog, R. (1992). Behavioral marital therapy for male alcoholics: Marital and drinking adjustment during the two years after treatment. *Behavior Therapy*, 23: 529-549.

O'Farrell, T., Cutter, H., & Floyd, F. (1985). Evaluating behavioral marital therapy for male alcoholics: Effects on marital adjustment and communication from before to after treatment. *Behavior Therapy*, 16: 147-167.

O'Farrell, T., & Fals-Stewart, W. (2000). Behavioral couples treatment for alcoholism and drug abuse. *Journal of Substance Abuse Treatment*, 18 (1) 51-54.

Orford, J. (1975). Alcoholism and marriage: The argument against specialism. *Journal of Studies on Alcohol*, 36 (11) 1537-1563.

Project COMBINE, Miller, W. (Primary Researcher) (1999). Sponsored by National Institute of Alcohol Abuse and Alcoholism.

Project MATCH Research Group (1993). Matching alcoholism treatments to client heterogeneity: Rationale and methods for a multi site clinical trial matching patients to alcoholism treatment. *Alcoholism: Clinical and Experimental Research*, 17 (6)1130-1145.

Project MATCH Research Group. (1997). Matching alcoholism treatment to client heterogeneity: Project MATCH post-treatment drinking outcomes. *Journal of Studies on Alcohol*, 58: 7-29.

Project MATCH Research Group. (1998). Matching alcoholism treatment to client heterogeneity: Treatment main effects and matching effects on drinking during treatment. *Journal of Studies on Alcohol*, 59: 631-639.

Sobell, M., Cunningham, J., & Sobell, L (1996). Recovery from alcohol problems with and without treatment: Prevalence in two population surveys. *American Journal of Public Health*, 86 (7) 996-972.

Sobell, M., Sobell, L., & Leo, G. (2000). Does enhanced social support improve outcomes for problem drinkers in guided self-change treatment? *Journal of Behavior Therapy & Experimental Psychiatry*, 31: 41-54.

Steinglass, P. (1976). Experimenting with family treatment approaches to alcoholism, 1950-1975: A review. *Family Process*, 15: 97-123.

Steinglass, P. (1981). The alcoholic family at home: Patterns of interaction in dry, wet, and transitional stages of alcoholism. *Archives of General Psychiatry*, 38: 578-584.

Steinglass, P., Davis, D., & Berenson, D. (1977). Observations of conjointly hospitalized alcoholic couples: Implications for theory and therapy. *Family Process*, 16: 1-16.

Vetere, A., & Henley, M. (2001). Integrating couples and family therapy into a community alcohol service: A pan-theoretical approach. *Journal of Family Therapy*, 23: 85-101.

Whelan, T. (1953). Wives of alcoholics: Four types observed in a family service agency. *Quarterly Journal of Studies on Alcohol*, 14: 632-641.

Zywiak, W., Longabaugh, R., & Wirtz, P. (2002). Decomposing the relationships between pretreatment social network characteristics and alcohol treatment outcome. *Journal of Studies on Alcohol*, 63: 114-121.

Young Children of Parents with Substance Use Disorders (SUD): A Review of the Literature and Implications for Social Work Practice

Neta Peleg-Oren
Meir Teichman

SUMMARY. This article reviews the scientific literature that focuses on school-age children of parents with substance use disorder (SUD). The review examined the subjects, instruments, and results of 10 scientific studies published from 1985 to the present (2005). Generally, school-age children of parents with SUD demonstrated a variety of emotional, cognitive, behavioral, and social problems. Specifically, (a) children of drug users (CODs) were at higher risk than children of alcoholics (COAs) for psychopathology and functional impairments, and (b) Children of parents diagnosed as having SUDs (particularly alcohol), along with anti-social personality disorder (ASPD) showed more negative psychosocial outcomes than children whose parents did

Neta Peleg-Oren, PhD, is Research Associate, Community-Based Intervention Research Group (CBIR-G), Florida International University, 11200 South West 8th Street, MARC 310, Miami, FL 33199.

Meir Teichman, PhD, is Professor, Bob Shapell School of Social Work, Tel-Aviv University, Tel-Aviv 69978, Israel (E-mail: teichma@post.tau.acc.il).

[Haworth co-indexing entry note]: "Young Children of Parents with Substance Use Disorders (SUD): A Review of the Literature and Implications for Social Work Practice." Peleg-Oren, Neta, and Meir Teichman. Co-published simultaneously in *Journal of Social Work Practice in the Addictions* (The Haworth Press, Inc.) Vol. 6, No. 1/2, 2006, pp. 49-61; and: *Impact of Substance Abuse on Children and Families: Research and Practice Implications* (ed: Shulamith Lala Ashenberg Straussner, and Christine Huff Fewell) The Haworth Press, Inc., 2006, pp. 49-61. Single or multiple copies of this article are available for a fee from The Haworth Document Delivery Service [1-800-HAWORTH, 9:00 a.m. - 5:00 p.m. (EST). E-mail address: docdelivery@haworthpress.com].

Available online at http://www.haworthpress.com/web/JSWPA
doi:10.1300/J160v06n01_03

not have ASPD. Recommendations for future research and implications for social work practice are discussed. *[Article copies available for a fee from The Haworth Document Delivery Service: 1-800-HAWORTH. E-mail address: <docdelivery@haworthpress.com> Website: <http://www.HaworthPress. com> © 2006 by The Haworth Press, Inc. All rights reserved.]*

KEYWORDS. Children of alcoholics, children of drug users, school-age children

INTRODUCTION

Growing with parents with SUD (Substance Use Disorders) has a considerable impact on the development of young children. During the last decade, the potentially negative impact of parental substance use has increasingly become of great concern to social policy decision-makers and practitioners alike (Barnard & McKeganey, 2004; Chassin, Carle, Nissim-Sabat, & Kumpfer, 2004; Jones, 2004; Teichman, 2001).

The present review examined relevant findings from scientific studies that focused on school-age children whose parents use alcohol and other illicit drugs. These studies were scientifically designed with appropriate control groups, and used reliable and valid instruments. The studies' focal points were the children's mental health, risks and/or protective factors, and psychosocial outcomes and consequences.

Developmental psychology literature indicates that early stages of life are fundamental to normal formation of personality, "ego identity," and secure attachment style. During this period of life children acquire their necessary social, and coping skills (Miller, 1993). These emotional, cognitive, social, and behavioral developmental processes take place in school, among peers, as well as in the family. Successful experiences provide the child with feelings of competence and mastery, whereas failure brings a sense of inadequacy and inferiority, low self esteem, and, in some cases, intergenerational transmission of substance abuse and other psychopathology (King & Chassin, 2004; Menuchin, 1987; Rodney & Mupier, 1999; Rydelius, 1997). Thus, for normal development, the child needs a safe and stable environment; a warm family that provides acceptance, trust, sense of autonomy, and security (Straussner, Weinstein, & Hernandez, 1979; Teichman & Kefir, 2000; Teichman & Teichman, 1990). A family, as we view it, is not just a sum of its individual members (mother, father, children, etc.), characteristics, and patterns of behavior, but a system that in which all members interact and affect each other (e.g., von Bertalanffy, 1968). Consequently, a dysfunctional parent may disrupt the ability of the family, as a whole, to provide the child, who is the most vulnerable member of the family, with the necessary resources to meet his or her needs (Teichman, Glaubman, & Garner, 1993). Furthermore, having a substance-abusing parent often results in the development of certain defense mechanisms and symptoms by children and adolescents (King & Chassin, 2004; Straussner et al., 1979). Despite the long-acknowledged importance of childhood developmental period in understanding the effects of parental substance use, only during the last decade has it been a focus of substantial systematic study. Prior to recent years, much of the work in this area stemmed from clinical observations and retrospective studies of adult children-of-parents with alcohol or drug abuse (ACOA/Ds). Moreover, due to nature of the subject-matter, few of the field studies were based on comparisons with a proper control group. Sher (1991) and other reviewers have noted a need for increased attention to lifespan developmental factors in considering the effects of parental substance use. Since an outcome at any particular time of assessment may differ depending on the current developmental level of the child, as well on many other factors (Seilhamer & Jacob, 1990; Sher, 1991; Windle & Searles, 1990), research on the psychosocial adjustment of children and adolescents in substance-abusing families cannot be automatically generalized (Harter, 2000).

The aim of this paper is to review scientifically sound published studies on children of parents with alcohol or illicit drug abuse (COA/Ds) that focus on the developmental period of childhood. We selected only studies in which the researchers investigated the psychosocial outcomes as measured by self-reports of the children. We assume that it is the child's own perception of her or his family at a given moment in life, rather than retrospective recollections of childhood experiences, that presents the most reliable picture of the impact of parental substance abuse on the child's development. Relying on memories and early recollections could raise doubts that parental substance use constitutes the dominant factor in the children's distress.

METHOD

This review is based on published studies abstracted in the following databases: PsychLit, Social Work Abstracts, Eric, and Medline. These four major databases were used in order to obtain the maximum number of referred publications in the field. In the present review, COA/Ds are defined as children (boys and girls) who have one or both parents that are addicted to alcohol or drugs and diagnosed as having SUD according to DSM-III or DSM-IV or any other reliable screening tests like: DIS (Diagnostic Interview Schedule), ICD-10, or MAST (Michigan Alcoholism Screening Test). "Childhood" in this review refers to elementary school-age children. We did not include adolescence period because even though adolescents are still living with their families, the physical and psychological changes that they are facing sometimes may influence their lives more than being children of parents with SUD. The review examines the target subjects, the instruments, and the results in each study.

RESULTS AND DISCUSSION

After using combinations of the terms "offspring/children of alcoholics," "offspring/children of drug abuse/use," "COAs, CODs, COA/Ds," "parental alcohol/drug abuse," "childhood," "school-age," we found only ten (10) papers published from 1985 up to the present (2005). As shown in Table 1, most of the studies investigated children of alcoholics (COAs). Children of parents with drug use disorders (CODs) were investigated only in comparison to COAs. Only two of the studies were longitudinal.

Results of the studies published since 1985 are consistent with the conclusions of previous reviews that found that school-age children of parents with SUD are at increased risk for negative outcomes in a number of dimensions: emotional, cognitive, behavioral, and social problems. Stress in families with substance use places the children at an increased risk for problems in their emotional development, including a relatively high level of depressive symptoms and anxiety, low self-esteem, guilt feelings, and loneliness (Reich, Earls, Frankel, & Shayka, 1993). Other studies suggested problems in cognitive development. According to Puttler et al. (1998), COAs had lower levels of intellectual functioning than non-COAs. Serious behavioral problems were found by Reich, Earls, Frankel, and Shayka (1993) and Kuperman, Schlosser, Lidral, and Reich (1999). Presumably, in such families, there are neither clear standards of behavior, nor limits or clear expectations. Parenting style is inconsistent: the same behavior of the child may be rewarded in one situation and be disciplined on another occasion. This may explain the findings of several studies that children of parents with SUD mani-

TABLE 1. Summary of Published Studies on COAD

Researchers	Subjects	Instruments	Results
Christozov & Toteva, 1989 (Longitudinal study)	220 COA 110 non-COA Aged 4-14	Developed questionnaires: 1. evaluated the child's mental status, attitudes towards the alcoholic father and the family, 2. evaluation of the alcoholic father	1. COA exhibited psychological problems such as fear, anxiety, low self-esteem, emotional deprivation, and aggressiveness compared to non-COA; 2. At follow-up COA demonstrated anti-social behavior.
Rubio-Stipec, Bird, Canino, Bravo, & Algria, 1991	Second stage–386 children of alcoholic parents and control group) Aged 4-16	DIS for the adult, CBCL, Clinical evaluation of the child, Scale adapted from the Coddington Life-Event Scale, Family APGAR Questionnaire, Developed question-naire for marital harmony, a measure of the physical status of the child, DISC, C-GAS.	1. Parental alcoholism in addition to creating an adverse family environment had an effect on the relative risk for maladjustment in the offspring; 2. The effects of parental alcoholism in children may not be different from the consequences of parental mental health.
Reich, Earls, Frankel, & Shayka, 1993	125 COA 158 control group Aged 6-18	For parents: HELPER, DICA-P, HEIC-P, CBCL. For Children: DICA, HEIC, PPVT, WRAT, CSEI. Also CBCL for teachers	COA exhibit high rate of psychopathology and may be at risk especially for oppositional and conduct disorder (CD) but not for depression.
Puttler, Zucker, Fitzgerald, & Bingham, 1998	44 children of antisocial alcoholic families, 94 children of non-antisocial alcoholic families, 74 children in control group Aged 3-8	For parents: family demographic questionnaire, SMAST, DIS, DDHQ, ASB, LAPS, CBCL. For children: WISC-R, Stanford-Binet, WRAT-R	1. COA had poorer functioning than control group; 2. Children from antisocial alcoholic families had greater problems than children from non-antisocial alcoholic families; 3. Boys had higher behavioral problems than girls in behavioral problems; 4. COA had lower levels of intellectual functioning than non-COA

TABLE 1 (continued)

Researchers	Subjects	Instruments	Results
Kuperman, Schlosser, Lidral, & Reich, 1999	266 COA 79 COA and anti-social behavior, 118 non-COA Average age 12	C-SSAGA	1. Parental alcoholism was associated with increased risks for ADHD, CD, and overanxious disorders; 2. Parental alcoholism plus ASPD was associated with increased risk for oppositional defiant disorder.
Moss, Baron, Hardie, & Vanyukov, 2001	70 COAD and Anti-Social Personality Disorder (ASPD) 268 COAD without ASPD 301 non-COAD/ASPD	SCID; K-SADS (Schizophrenia); SCID-II	COAD+ASPD showed more major depression, conduct disorder, ADHD, oppositional defiant disorder, separation anxiety disorder, and higher internalizing and externalizing behavior problems compared to other groups
Peleg-Oren, 2001	72 COAD 76 non-COAD Aged 8-11	For parent: family socio-demographic questionnaire, ASFS. For children: CRPBI, FACESIII (only cohesion), ASCQ, EDS	1. No significant differences were found between the two groups in family cohesion, parenting styles, and psychosocial adjustment; 2. Insecure-avoidant attachment style was more prevalent among COAD than among non-COAD.
Wilens, Biederman, Bredin, Hahesy, Abrantes et al., 2002	22 COA 22 COD (opiod dependence) 139 control group Aged 6-18	SCID; KSADS-E (epidemic version–childhood disorders); Wide Range Achievement Test–WRAT; WISC-R; Social Adjustment Inventory–SAICA; Moos FES.	1. The COD (opioid dependence) had more psychopathology and functional impairment that the COA; 2. COAD were of lower SES, had significantly more difficulties in academic, social, and family functioning, and higher rates of psychopathology than non-COAD.

54

Study	Sample	Measures	Findings
Kelley & Fals-Stewart, 2004	COD COA or non-SA fathers Aged 8-12	For children: K-SADS-PL. For parents: SCID, TLFB, PSC.	COD were more likely to have a lifetime psychiatric diagnosis; COD were more than twice as likely to exhibit clinical levels of behavioral symptoms.
Werner & Johnson, 2004 (Longitudinal study)	65 COA–aged 2 at beginning phase over 30 years	Aged 1,2,10–Observation by social workers and nurses; Grade 4-5–Behavior evaluation by teachers. Grade 8,10,12–Scholastic Aptitude & Achievement tests. Age 10–Parents' interview Aged 18–Child's interview Age 18,31,31–Rotter LCS, perceived stress and support questionnaires Age 31, 32–EAS Score on California Psychological Inventory & Nowicki. Information from Court and Dept. of Mental Health	COA who became competent adults relied on significantly larger numbers of sources of support in their childhood.

fested problem behaviors as early as pre-school age (Kuperman et al., 1999; Puttler, Zucker, Fitzgerald, & Bingham, 1998). Furthermore, parents who had anti-social or conduct disorder diagnosis in addition to SUD further affected their children. Indeed, children of parents with SUD and anti-social personality disorder (ASPD) had even greater problems than offspring of non-ASPD alcoholic families (Moss, Baron, Hardie, & Vanyukov, 2001; Puttler et al., 1998). Two studies that compared the psychopathology of COAs to CODs indicate that CODs exhibited more psychological problems such as fear, anxiety, low self-esteem, emotional deprivation, and aggressiveness than COAs or non-COAs (Kelley & Fals-Stewart, 2004; Wilens, Biederman, Bredin, Hahesy, Abrantes et al., 2002).

Either as a result of these problems, or as an independent issue, several studies pointed out setbacks in the COAs' social development: These children were frequently described as reticent and reserved and their social life limited (Christov & Toteva, 1989; Rubio-Stipec, Bird, Canino, Bravo, & Algria, 1991). According to these studies, shame and secrecy were the main reasons for the social isolation.

However, contrary to these findings, Peleg-Oren (2001) did not find differences between children of addicted fathers and their matched controls. Peleg-Oren investigated children, 8 to 11 years old, whose fathers were diagnosed as having SUD. They were matched with same gender/age children attending the same school and residing in the same neighborhood. Their self reports of their parents' parenting styles and family cohesion were compared as well as their psychosocial adjustment. Contrary to previously reviewed studies, no significant differences were found between the COA/Ds and non-COA/Ds in family cohesion, parenting styles, psychosocial adjustment, and emotional distress.

Finally, longitudinal studies provide us with knowledge about the long-term effects of growing up with parents with SUD; to what extent such an experience is perceived as a traumatic one, and how such experiences affect the course of development from childhood to adolescence, and, thereafter, to adulthood. Only two longitudinal studies are reported. These studies provided support to the commonly accepted assumption that parental SUD entails life-long developmental negative repercussions for those children. Children of COA/Ds experienced social-emotional difficulties and problems as early as infancy due to dysfunctional life experiences with parents with SUD. However, Werner and Johnson (2004), whose longitudinal study followed children of alcoholics from the age of 2 years for over a 30-year period, challenged these sweeping conclusions. They reported that the availability of support systems significantly affected the development of the children into adulthood. Availability of support systems within the extended family or in the community may have a positive influence on the child's ability to cope effectively with the trauma of growing up in such families. Factors such as strong extended family support and the maintenance of family routines were important mediating factors on the potential for positive outcomes for the child (Barnard, 2003; Barnard & McKeganey, 2004).

This brief view of the literature highlights the importance of studying risk and protective factors in the life of a child growing with parents with SUD. Garbarino (1999) defined resilience as the ability to bounce back from crisis and overcome stress and injury, and as a mean of developing a positive sense of self. Dawe, Harnett, Staiger, and Dadds (2000) pointed out that the likelihood of developing psychosocial problems is not determined by one single risk factor (like parental SUD), but by interactions among risk and protective factors over time. Protective factors enable the child's healthy growth and development. Teit and Huizinga (2002) summarized this in stating that: "Many studies have found that numerous high-risk individuals defy unfavorable outcomes."

LIMITATIONS OF THE STUDY

The limitations of this review must be considered. Even though the studies used reliable instruments, it was very hard to directly compare the studies due to the incompatibility of the instruments. In addition, this review included only English and Hebrew language studies published over two decades, and included only papers in journals abstracted in the previously discussed databases. Scientific studies published in other languages and/or not abstracted in those databases might be of great importance in terms of culture diversity.

IMPLICATIONS FOR SOCIAL WORK PRACTICE

Findings from the present review can be used to improve decision making about intervention. First, although COA/Ds are at high-risk for negative psychosocial consequence, it is a heterogeneous population with diverse developmental needs. Evaluation of the needs and resources of the family and the children is vital in order to plan and implement effective and appropriate interventions for the children and for the family. Secondly, due to the obstacles to effectively implementing interventions in real-world social work practice settings with potentially limited resources, social workers must take into consideration two significant issues: (a) In most cases, CODs (opioid) are at higher risk than COAs (alcohol) for psychopathology and functional impairments; (b) Parental SUD (particularly alcohol) in addition to anti-social personality disorder is associated with more negative psychosocial outcomes to the child than parental substance use without ASPD. Hence, we recommend that:

- High-risk CODs should have priority in assessment and intervention than COAs;
- There is an urgent need to identify COAs from families where anti-social behavior is evident due to the intergenerational transmission of the disorder, and to develop early intervention programs that address their needs;
- Comprehensive intervention programs should consider both the family and the children, as well as members of the extended family, who may provide support for the child and for the non-addicted spouse (e.g., Aviram & Spitz, 2003; Barnard & McKeganey, 2004; Csiernik, 2002).

School-age children of parents with SUD are rarely the direct focus of intervention. This stems from the assumption that children will indirectly benefit from the assistance offered to their parents (Miller, 2003). Nevertheless, during the last decade several experimental interventions with children of parents with SUD have been designed and implemented (i.e., Peleg-Oren, 2002a). Group intervention is one of the remedial tools that are appropriate to the developmental stage of elementary school-age children. At this stage peer-group becomes important to them. The group can provide a support and an arena where social skills are developed; the group offers the child the possibility of belonging and of sharing their burden with other children suffering from similar dysfunctional family situations (Peleg-Oren, 2002b).

CONCLUSION

More research is needed to examine the risk and protective factors associated with the intergenerational transmission of substance use. In particular, future research should look closely at critical points in time in the developmental process identifying the trajectory of functional impairments and substance use among children of parents with SUD. Given that these children are at high risk to develop SUD and other mental health problems as adolescents and adults, the development of innovative intervention programs for the children should be the main concern.

REFERENCES

Aviram, R.B., & Spitz, H.I. (2003). Substance abuse couple therapy: Clinical considerations and relational themes. *Journal of Family Psychotherapy*, 14(3), 1-18.

Barnard, M. (2003). Between a rock and a hard place: The role of relatives in protecting children from the effects of parental drug problems. *Child & Family Social Work*, 8 (4), 291-299

Barnard, M., & McKeganey, N. (2004). The impact of parental problem drug use on children: What is the problem and what can be done to help? *Addiction*, 99, 552-559.

Bertalanffy, K.L. von, (1968). *General Systems Theory*. NY: Braziller.

Carle, A.C., & Chassin, L. (2004). Resilience in a community sample of children of alcoholics: Its prevalence and relation to internalizing symptomatology and positive affect. *Journal of Applied Developmental Psychology*, 25(5), 577-595.

Chassin, L., Carle, A.C., Nissim-Sabat, D., & Kumpfer, K.L. (2004). Fostering Resilience in Children of Alcoholic Parents. In K.I. Maton, C.J. Schellenbach, B. J. Leadbeater, and A. L. Solarz (Ed.). *Investigating in Children, Youth, Families, and communities: Strengths-Based Research and Policy* (pp. 137-155). Washington, DC: American Psychological Association.

Christozov, C., & Toteva, S. (1989). Abuse and neglect of children brought up in families with an alcoholic father in Bulgaria. *Child Abuse & Neglect*, 13, 153-155.

Clark, D.B. (2004). The nature history of adolescent alcohol use disorders. *Addiction*, 99 (suppl. 2), 5-22.

Csiernik, N. (2002). Counseling for the family: The neglected aspect of addiction treatment in Canada. *Journal of Social Work Practice in the Addictions*, 2(1), 79-92.

Dawe, S., Harnett, P.H., Staiger, P., & Dadds, M.R.(2000). Parental training skills and methadone maintanance: clinical opportunities and challenges. *Drug & Alcohol Dependence*, 60, 1-11.

Garbarino, J. (1999). *Lost boys: Why our sons turn violent and how can we save them?* New York: Free Press.

Harter, L.H. (2000). Psychosocial adjustment of adult children of alcoholics: A review of the recent empirical literature. *Clinical Psychology Review*, 20(3), 311-337.

Jones, L. (2004). The prevalence and characteristics of substance abusers in a child protective service sample. *Journal of Social Work Practice in the Addictions*, 4(2), 33-50.

Kelley, M.L., & Fals-Stewart, W. (2004). Psychiatric disorders of children living with drug-abusing, alcohol-abusing, and non substance-abusing fathers. *Journal of the American Academy of Child & Adolescent Psychiatry*, 43(5), 621-628.

King, K.M., & Chassin, L. (2004). Mediating and moderated effects of adolescent behavioral under control and parenting in the prediction of drug use disorders in
emerging adulthood. *Psychology of Addictive Behaviors, 18*, 239-249.

Kuperman, S., Schlosser, S.S., Lidral, J., & Reich, W. (1999). Relationship of child
psychopathology to parental alcoholism and antisocial personality disorder. *Journal
of the American Academy of Child and Adolescent Psychiatry*, 38(6), 686-692.

Minuchin, S. (1987). My many voices. In J.K. Zeig (Ed.). *The evolution of psychotherapy*. New York: Brunner/Mazel, pp. 5-13.

Miller, P.H. (1993). *Theories of Developmental Psychology*. New York: W.H. Freeman
and Company.

Miller, W.R. (2003). A collaborative approach to working with families. *Addiction*, 98, 5-6.

Moss, H.B., Baron, D.A., Hardie, T.L., & Vanyukov, M.M. (2001). Preadolescent children of substance-dependent fathers with antisocial personality disorder: Psychiatric
disorders and problem behaviors. *American Journal on Addiction*, 10(3), 269-278.

Peleg-Oren, N. (2001). *Children of addicted fathers: Family resources, attachment
style, emotional, and social adjustment.* Unpublished PhD Thesis, Tel-Aviv University, Faculty of Social Science, Ramat-Aviv, Israel (in Hebrew).

Peleg-Oren, N. (2002a). Drugs–Not Here! Model of group intervention as preventive
therapeutic tool for children of drug addicts. *Journal of Drug Education, 32*(3),
245-259.

Peleg-Oren, N. (2002b). Group intervention for children of drug-addicted parents using expressive techniques. *Clinical Social Work Journal*, 30, 403-418.

Puttler, L.I., Zucker, R.A., Fitzgerald, H.E., & Bingham, C.R. (1998). Behavioral outcomes among children of alcoholics during the early and middle years: Familial subtype variations. *Alcoholism: Clinical and Experimental Research*, 22(9), 1962-1972.

Reich, W., Earls, F., Frankel, O., & Shayka, J.J. (1993). Psychopathology in children of
alcoholics. *Journal of the American Academy of Child and Adolescent Psychiatry*, 32
(5), 995-1002.

Rodney, H.E., & Mupier, R. (1999). Impact of parental alcoholism on self-esteem and
depression among African-American adolescents. *Journal of Child & Adolescent
Substance Abuse*, 8, 55-71.

Rydelius, P.A. (1997). Annotation: Are children of alcoholics a clinical concern for child
and adolescent psychiatrists of today? *Journal of Child Psychology & Psychiatry &
Allied Disciplines*, 38(6), 615-624

Rubio-Stipec, M., Bird, H., Canino, G., Bravo, M., & Alegria, M. (1991). Children of alcoholic parents in the community, *Journal of Studies on Alcohol*, 52(1), 78-88.

Seilhamer, R.A., & Jacob, T. (1990). Family factors and adjustment of children of alcoholics. In: M. Windle, & J.S. Searles (Eds.), *Children of alcoholics: Critical perspectives* (pp. 168-186). New York: Guilford Press.

Sher, K.J. (1991). *Children of alcoholics: A critical appraisal of theory and research.*
Chicago: University of Chicago Press.

Straussner, S.L.A., Weinstein, D.L., & Hernandez, R. (1979). Effects of alcoholism on
the family system. *Health & Social Work*, 4(4), 111-127.

Teichman, M. (2001). *Alcohol and alcoholism: Causes, prevention, and intervention.*
Tel-Aviv: Tel-Aviv University: Ramot Publishing House. (In Hebrew).

Teichman, M., Glaubman, H., & Garner, M. (1993). From preadolescence to middle age adulthood: The perceived need for interpersonal resources in four developmental phases. In U.G. Foa, J.M. Converse, K. Torenblom, & E.B. Foa (Eds.), *Resource Theory: Explorations and Applications*, 157-165. New York: Academic Press.

Teichman, M., & Kefir, E. (2000). The effects of perceived parental behaviors, attitudes, and substance-use on adolescent attitudes toward and intent to use psychoactive substances. *Journal of Drug Education*, 30, 191-202.

Teichman, Y., & Teichman, M. (1990). Interactional view of depression: Review and integration. *Journal of Family Psychology*, 3, 349-367.

Tiet, Q., & Huizinga, D. (2002). Dimensions of the construct of resilience and adaptation among inner-city youth. *Journal of Adolescent Research,* 17, 260-276.

Werner, E.E., & Johnson, J.L. (2004). The role of caring adults in the lives of children of alcoholics. *Substance Use and Misuse*, 39 (5), 699-720.

Wilens, T.E., Biederman, J., Bredin, E., Hahesy, A.L., Abrantes, A., Neft, D., Millstein, R., & Spencer, T.J. (2002). A family study of the high-risk children of opioid-and alcohol-dependent parents. *American Journal on Addiction*, 11 (1), 41-51.

Windle, M., & Searles, J.S. (1990). Summary, integration, and future directions: Toward a life-span perspective. In M. Windle, & J.S. Searles (Eds.), *Children of alcoholics: Critical perspectives.* (pp. 217-238). New York: Guilford Press.

The Impact of Methamphetamine Use
on Parenting

Julie A. Brown
Melinda Hohman

SUMMARY. Children whose parents abuse substances are often exposed to chaotic and neglectful lifestyles. Because of the increase in methamphetamine abuse, especially by females of child-bearing age, it is important to understand how the use of this drug impacts parenting. In this qualitative study, ten parents being treated for methamphetamine abuse were interviewed. Results indicated that while using, parents utilized a polarized style of parenting and specific drug management strategies, allowed exposure to violence, created upheaval in their children's daily living structure, and felt ambivalence when discussing these effects on children. Implications for social work practice include early intervention focusing on strengthening parenting skills. *[Article copies available for a fee from The Haworth Document Delivery Service: 1-800-HAWORTH. E-mail address: <docdelivery@haworthpress.com> Website: <http://www.HaworthPress. com> © 2006 by The Haworth Press, Inc. All rights reserved.]*

Julie A. Brown, ACSW, is Counselor, Home Based Services, New Alternatives, Incorporated, San Diego, CA.

Melinda Hohman, PhD, is Professor, San Diego State University School of Social Work, 5500 Campanile Drive, San Diego, CA 92182-4119 (E-mail: mhohman@mail. sdsu.edu).

[Haworth co-indexing entry note]: "The Impact of Methamphetamine Use on Parenting." Brown, Julie A., and Melinda Hohman. Co-published simultaneously in *Journal of Social Work Practice in the Addictions* (The Haworth Press, Inc.) Vol. 6, No. 1/2, 2006, pp. 63-88; and: *Impact of Substance Abuse on Children and Families: Research and Practice Implications* (ed: Shulamith Lala Ashenberg Straussner, and Christine Huff Fewell) The Haworth Press, Inc., 2006, pp. 63-88. Single or multiple copies of this article are available for a fee from The Haworth Document Delivery Service [1-800-HAWORTH, 9:00 a.m. - 5:00 p.m. (EST). E-mail address: docdelivery@haworthpress.com].

Availlable online at http://www.haworthpress.com/web/JSWPA
doi:10.1300/J160v06n01_04

63

KEYWORDS: Methamphetamines, impact on parenting, drug abuse

INTRODUCTION

The last decade has seen an increase in methamphetamine use in the United States by both males and females and a concomitant increase in clients entering alcohol and other drug (AOD) treatment programs who report methamphetamine as their primary drug (Community Epidemiology Work Group, 2000; Hohman & Clapp, 1999; SAMHSA, 2001). The problem has grown especially among females in their childbearing years (Cretzmeyer, Sarrazin, Huber, Block, & Hall, 2003; Gorman, Clark, Nelson, Applegate, Amato, & Scrol, 2003; National Institute of Justice, 1999; Reiber, Galloway, Cohen, Hsu, & Lord, 2000). Between 1997 and 1999, 11,300 women who were admitted to public AOD treatment centers in San Diego cited methamphetamine as their primary drug. They had an average of 1.5 children under the age of 18, representing 16,950 children (Hohman, Shillington, & Clapp, 2002).

Social workers report that children of methamphetamine users are often neglected, and that they have found infants and children with unchanged diapers, in dirty housing, with no food or formula, and with dirty syringes that were easily accessible. Children of parents who use methamphetamine may not only be affected by their parents' drug usage, but also from the home manufacturing of the drug. Living in a home where there is manufacturing often exposes children to the toxic chemicals and fumes, with the potential for lung damage, fire or explosion. Children living in such environment have tested positive for methamphetamine exposure (Ells, Sturgis, & Wright, 2002; Hohman, Oliver, & Wright, 2004).

In terms of their interactions with their children, parents who abuse various substances have been found to have inconsistent and inappropriate emotional responsiveness and to be unpredictable and impulsive (Beebe & Walley, 1995; Greif & Drechsler, 1993; Hogan, 1998; Mayes, 1995). Methamphetamine abusers may also become paranoid, delusional, live a disorganized lifestyle, and experience interpersonal violence (Cohen et al., 2003; Cretzmeyer et al., 2003). Consequently, their children may experience a compromised sense of security and an inability to continuously rely on their parents for their basic needs (Ells, Sturgis, & Wright, 2002; Hohman, Oliver, & Wright, 2004). No studies, to date, have investigated the relationship between methamphetamine abuse and parenting.

LITERATURE REVIEW

Methamphetamine is a stimulant in the same category as cocaine, and provides euphoria, alertness, and a sense of well-being. It is usually sold as a powder that can be ingested orally, smoked, snorted, or injected. Unlike cocaine, the drug is metabolized at a much slower rate, thus its effects can last from six to eight hours. Negative effects from the drug include increased heart rate, stomach cramps, anxiety, paranoia, and hallucinations (Anglin, Burke, Perrochet, Stamper, & Dawud-Noursi, 2000; Rawson, 1999; Wermuth, 2000). Users tend to use excessively over time, exhibiting stereotypic or repetitive behavior during binge use. For example, a user may excessively clean an apartment or disassemble and assemble a computer. Binges may last from several days to a week without sleep, with users crashing and sleeping for 12-18 hours during withdrawal. Withdrawal can also be marked by intense depression and irritability (Murray, 1998).

Children living in homes with parents who use methamphetamine may be at risk for neglect due to the binge/crash cycle, as well as other effects from adults' use of the drug (Stalkup, 2000). Methamphetamine use has also been linked with violent and aggressive behavior, including domestic violence and violence inherent in drug trafficking (Brecht, O'Brien, von Mayrhauser, & Anglin, 2004; Cohen et al., 2003). Parents may also have many sexual partners as methamphetamine use also enhances the libido (Gibson, Leamon, & Flynn, 2002). Because methamphetamine can be manufactured at home, using recipes from the Internet, children living in these homes are placed at an increased risk of exposure to chemicals and possible explosions (Hohman et al., 2004; Irvine & Chin, 1997).

While there have been no studies to date regarding the impact of methamphetamine use on parenting, researchers have investigated the effects of other substance use on parenting. Miller, Smyth, and Mudar (1999) interviewed women (n = 170) recruited from treatment programs, drunk driver classes, domestic violence shelters, and also through random households. Mothers who had abused substances as well as experienced parental and domestic violence were found to display higher levels of punitiveness toward their children, even while in recovery, as compared to those who had no history of AOD problems.

Hardesty and Black (1999) interviewed 20 Puerto Rican cocaine and/or heroin users who were also mothers. They believed that they had maintained certain standards of childcare while using drugs, and that their children served as sources of motivation to recover. Maintaining standards for their mothering not only ensured that their children were taken care of, it also helped to preserve their self-esteem. Believing that they were "good mothers" and keeping that role central, became what the authors call a lifeline into, through, and out of addiction.

Several studies have investigated parenting practices of clients in methadone clinics. Nurco, Blatchley, Hanlon, O'Grady, and McCarren (1998) analyzed parental functioning in 313 clients (79% female) in methadone maintenance programs. Respondents were asked to describe their childhood experiences as children of addicts, as well as to describe their own current parenting practices as addicts themselves. Results indicated three primary findings: that perception of stability is dependent on the maternal presence, that participants reported higher levels of functioning than their parents, and that male alcoholism was overwhelmingly present in families with drug problems.

Greif and Dreschler (1993) described themes that emerged from a parenting group at a methadone program. Mothers and fathers described chaos and inconsistency in their parenting, both while using heroin and on methadone, as well as guilt from neglecting their children in the past. Difficult relationships with their own parents impacted parenting.

Another study of mothers in methadone treatment found that they were more likely to leave their children with relatives than a comparison group of non-drug using mothers living in the same area (Suchman & Luthar, 2000). This was an effort to protect them from their chaotic lifestyles. Additionally, both groups of parents were found to be equally authoritarian, which researchers suggested was also adaptive behavior for parents who raise children in low-income and dangerous environments.

PURPOSE OF THE STUDY

The purpose of this study was to understand the specific impact of methamphetamine addiction on parenting skills, and inevitably, on the involved children. The hope is to build knowledge in order to enhance treatment services for parents and their children. Research questions for this study were:

1. How did participants' methamphetamine use affect the role of parenting?

2. As their methamphetamine use increased, how did parents' roles, standards, and abilities to handle daily stress change over time?
3. How did parents manage their use or compensate for it with their children?
4. How did parents experience and respond to their children while they were using?
5. How did methamphetamine use affect family dynamics?

METHOD AND PARTICIPANTS

Because little is known about the impact of methamphetamine use on parenting and family dynamics, this qualitative study used in-depth interviewing to allow participants to tell their stories. This allowed for exploration of common concerns and themes regarding this problem.

Participants were recruited from a publicly funded out-patient alcohol and other drug (AOD) treatment program located in San Diego, California. Most clients attending this program have been court-ordered to attend treatment, either as a deterrent from more jail time or as an incentive to regain custody of their children; many were actively involved with Child Protective Services (CPS). One main requirement for treatment eligibility was that the client is parenting a child under the age of 18, though the majority of clients did not have custody of their children (Brown, 2001).

Clients were recruited by the first author, who attended two separate "community meetings" at the agency, which are mandatory meetings held once a week for both day and evening clients and staff. After explaining the purpose of the study, as well as the general participation guidelines, provisions established to insure confidentiality were described. This included a reference to the Certificate of Confidentiality, which had been obtained from the National Institute of Drug Abuse. Due to the nature of the questions to be posed and the material discussed, permission to conduct the study was granted only if the Certificate of Confidentiality was obtained. The Certificate offers protection to both study participants and researchers collecting information that, if disclosed, could have adverse consequences on the personal lives of the participants. It ensures that researchers or anyone else with access to the collected data can refuse to disclose it in response to any request, from the federal to the local level, even in a court of law (*http://grants1.nih. gov/grants/policy/coc/*). It is hoped that with such protection participants will feel more comfortable and more willing to disclose information for the purpose of research studies. Clients were also assured that participation in the study was completely voluntary even if they were court-ordered to attend treatment. They were also encouraged to mention the study to peers not in the program who had used methamphetamine while parenting. Additionally, flyers were posted in both the cafeteria and front waiting area indicating a need for interested volunteers to discuss "methamphetamine and parenting issues" for not more than one hour. Agency counselors were also given extra flyers to give to any client whom they thought might qualify. Potential participants were asked to contact the first author by phone or by a note left at the agency for her. An incentive of two movie passes was offered for participation.

A total of 32 clients at the community meetings expressed interest in participating in the study. Clients who volunteered were individually prescreened; subsequently, eight had to be removed from the list due to the fact that methamphetamine was not their primary drug of choice and/or they had given insufficient contact information. Of the remaining 24 individuals, 10 methamphetamine users who were diverse in race, ethnicity, and gender were chosen to be interviewed.

DATA COLLECTION AND MEASURES

Interviews took place at either a vacant counseling office or the conference room of the agency at an appointed time scheduled specifically for this purpose. The participants were given the Consent to Act as a Research Subject and the Informed Consent to review and sign or verbally agreed to the terms. Each was given a copy of the signed form. Participants were also asked to give a first name that would be used throughout the study (from labeling the audiotapes to the final compilation of information). The tapes and notepaper were then labeled as such in the client's presence. The interviews were audiotaped and additional notes were taken for the purpose of clarification. The conversations lasted between 45 minutes and one hour.

At the end of the interview, participants were thanked and given the movie passes as compensation. All of the paperwork involved in the above-mentioned procedures was kept in a locked, transportable file accessible only to the authors.

The semi-structured interview was divided into three parts. First, the participants were asked demographic questions about themselves, their children (ages and places of residence) and how they came to be clients at the agency. Next, they were asked about the initiation and progression of their methamphetamine use, including the logistics of using and storing the drugs and paraphernalia around their children. The assumption was that methamphetamine use affects one's judgment, family dynamics, the home environment and specifically, the relationships between children and the using parents. To that end, questions included, "How did you respond to your children when you were high, tweaking, or coming down from your use?" and "Do you think you were able to handle your role as a parent while you were using?" Finally, the participants were asked to describe what the relationships with their partners were like while they were using. We also inquired as to their positive behaviors with their children.

ANALYSIS

A professional typist transcribed the audiotapes. The transcriptionist noted areas of the interview that had been inaudible or unclear; these gaps were subsequently filled through the use of the additional notes that had been made during the interview process (Padgett, 1998). Each transcript was read to note emerging themes, concerns and phrases that had been presented by the participants. These were coded using an open-ended approach (no prior formulated concepts) in a line-by-line analysis into category names. Additional readings of the transcripts and categories were refined and reorganized as specific themes emerged. Memos were written to conceptualize and categorize these themes and concerns. The transcripts were then reread to determine that they were coded with these themes (Padgett, 1998). Representative quotes were subsequently pulled from each theme (Miles & Huberman, 1984; Padgett, 1998; Tutty, Rothery, & Grinnell, 1996).

RESULTS

All of the participants in this study were current clients of a public treatment agency and identified their primary problem drug as methamphetamine. In some cases, counselors or friends had referred them to treatment; however, eight of the 10 of the participants were involved with Child Protective Services, and three had served time in jail. Four participants were Hispanic, four were Caucasian, and two were African-American. Three were males. The participants' time in recovery ranged from 2 months to 3 1/2 years; the average recovery time was 16 months. Participants' ages ranged from 24 to 45 years old. The ten parents had a total of 40 children, however at the time of the interview, only 17 of these 40 children were living with them. Eighteen children were either in foster or kinship care, or had been adopted; the whereabouts of two of the children were unknown. Three of the children were over 18 years old and living on their own. The 17 children ranged in age from eight months to 17 years old; the average age was eight years old.

COMMON THEMES:
BEHAVIOR, BELIEFS, AND OUTCOMES

Upon reading, rereading, and coding each transcribed interview, six common themes regarding the impact of methamphetamine use on parenting became apparent. They are listed and defined in Figure 1: (a) Polar Parenting; (b) Drug Management; (c) The Separate Life; (d) Domestic Violence; (e) The Effect on the Children; and (f) Retrospective Ambivalence.

Theme 1: Polar Parenting

As the conversations began, it quickly became clear that, according to these parents, during their drug use they had often exhibited quite polarized styles of expression toward their children. Extreme feelings of anger or apathy appeared to be typical, but these were not balanced out with expressions of interest, joy, or even peace. Emotionally, there

FIGURE 1. Themes Regarding the Impact of Methamphetamine Use on Parenting

1.	Polar Parenting	extreme feelings of anger or apathy
2.	Drug Management	the logistics of using methamphetamine as a parent of young children
3.	The Separate Life	parents removing themselves, and their drug use, from their children
4.	Domestic Violence	violence between marital and live-in partners, as well as violent crimes against family members in the home
5.	Effects on Children	physical, environmental, emotional, and psychological impacts
6.	Retrospective Ambivalence	differing opinions and beliefs about whether or not they were able to handle their roles as parents while using methamphetamine

did not seem to be a consistent "middle ground." According to the participants, developmentally appropriate child behaviors, milestones, and expressions of feelings were often either ignored or not tolerated. Questions posed specifically to learn about their reactions to the children's times of laughter and celebration yielded answers indicating antithetical feelings or behavior:

> Cheryl: One time he was proud, showing his report card and I was "Oh, what's it going to be? All F's?" I just was so negative about him all the time.

> Steve: I kind of remember Christmas and birthdays, [but eventually] I had to hide in the bedroom because I just couldn't function.

> Barbara: I didn't have any of those [holidays, etc.]. I pretty much became really cold, really bitter, got away from it as much as I could, to the point to where she was taken away from me. If she was happy I was like ok, honey, go play with your friends now. I just, you know, I didn't give a shit.

> Molly: I would get irritable and crabby sometimes. Sometimes I'd get wild, I'd want to dance with them or just have a good time . . . but then I would sleep a lot.

Avoidance and apathy were manifested in a different ways. Many described locking themselves in the bedroom or bathroom, not just to use, but also to get away from their children. Sleeping is a side effect from coming down, so the parents would often need to sleep excessively. This was difficult to do when the children were needy, boisterous, or simply interested in spending time with their parent. Some would tell their children that they felt ill, or were tired. One woman recalled that she often employed the older son as the babysitter, and would ask him to take the younger one out of the house so she could use drugs, or come down without disruption. Others reported becoming overly permissive just to keep their children away from them, even when they were high:

> Barbara: She's at the door, "Mommy, Mommy," you know, and I'd tell her to go away or something.

Cheryl: When I was high, I was more, "Do what you want." My child would ask to go somewhere . . . I never investigated where they were going. I didn't care if there was a big [traffic] intersection or not, I'd say "okay, yeah go ahead."

Most participants were able to give some examples of how they physically took care of their children. For example, meals were made either by themselves or another family member, and they could recall that at times their homes were clean (especially when they were high and full of energy). Emotional attendance to the children seemed to be quite challenging, however, and they described being angry and cranky:

Donna: I was in a bad mood. They knew that, it was like, because I was tired. My temper was really, really bad where I would get up and start throwing things. That's when they stayed away from me . . . I'd be dozing in and out of sleep. You know, you don't want anybody to know that you're coming down, so you're trying to stay awake and sleep at the same time.

Cheryl: And I'd call him names. They'd keep bugging, so eventually I'd be like, "Hey, you little son of a bitch . . . "

Theme II: Drug Management

Asking the participants about where they hid their methamphetamine and drug paraphernalia initially seemed to be a relatively easy question to answer. They were all quick to respond. Some kept it on themselves, stuffed in a bra or pocket. Many described using hiding places, and only one participant admitted to leaving a pipe within reach of a minor. Kitchen drawers, canisters, and even electrical outlets and vents were used to store the drugs. Creativity in storage served two purposes:

Cheryl: Those cardboard paper towel things, I'd wrap it in a paper towel, stick everything inside and then stick it like underneath my mattress or something. So that way the mattress wouldn't crush the pipe . . . and the kids won't find it.

Molly: I'd roll it up in a tissue in a sock, at the bottom of the dirty clothes pile where I know that nobody was gonna go. Or I'd have my clothes hung up, and I'd put it in the inside pocket. Nobody was trying on my clothes . . .

There was clearly some forethought in how they would store and use the methamphetamine. As we continued to explore this area, some participants offered their philosophies regarding their children and drug use. Several parents emphasized that they had made somewhat concerted efforts to keep their children away from the drugs, and vice versa. One woman would use in another room, with the door closed, so the smoke would not affect her child. Another would only use when her children were at school, or after they fell asleep at night. One woman claimed that she maintained abstinence while she was pregnant and later while she was nursing, so that her children would not be drug-exposed:

Ally: My one child I only nursed for a few months, so I could go back to getting high.

Steve: You know, since I had the kids, it wasn't like I needed to be like having things laying around, you know what I'm saying? I was a little dopey now, but I was also a little smart. I've seen enough TV where kids [get hurt by drug use]. I have an awareness, so I never left things laying around.

Asking for more detail resulted in curtailed answers. During the conversations, we had begun to explore if logistically an actively using parent could always keep the drugs away from their children. One participant commented that she realized that indeed, even though she smoked in a closed room, eventually opening the door released the fumes onto her waiting children. One father discussed having to bring his children on a drug run:

(Q: "Were your kids ever with you when you went to get drugs or deal?")

Dario: I'm not going to say never, okay, but I'm going to say hardly ever. Well, I mean I guess I would say they've never been with me to deal drugs. They've been with me, you know, like I'm coming down and I need a pick me up and I just stop by somebody's house to pick up a little bit.

(Q: "When you went to somebody's house, did they walk with you into the house? Were they in the car?")

Dario: They've been in the house.

(Q: "Okay. Did you have them stay in the same room?")

Dario: Absolutely not.

One mother "kept her kids safe" another way–she repeatedly left them in crowded, child-friendly but public areas while she went to procure more methamphetamine. She believed that dropping them off would keep them busy. She also thought that it ensured that if she was hurt or even killed, there would be people around to take care of them.

Cheryl: In the back of my mind I still thought about them in a way, you know.

(Q: "Did you tell your kids you were leaving them there or did they not know?")

Cheryl: At first I told them I was going to stay away for awhile . . . And then I tracked [the oldest one, the 10 year-old] back down and told her I'd be right back. And she doesn't want me to go. [She said], "Mom, can you stay? When are you coming back?" I said I'll be back in about 15 minutes . . . I was gone for hours.

Theme III: The Separate Life

Typically, the parent's intention was to keep the children separate from the "world of drugs." Each parent noted that at some point in time, there was a conscious effort to either hide their methamphetamine from their children, or to remove the children from the situation. Another method was to literally remove themselves, the parents, from their children:

Warren: I'd come back in the morning, in time to go to work. The wife dropped the kids off [to school] in the morning and I'd pick them up in the afternoon. It was a lot less parenting, which is really sad. I was taking off when I was high like that. I preferred to be with them when I was sober . . . I wouldn't have my children endangered by being around drugs, have drugs, or having people bring drugs over, or have them in the car with me on drugs. I wouldn't have none of that. That was separate.

Marta: I wouldn't come home. I kept [my daughter] away with my family. I wouldn't come home during the time when I was coming down. I would come home when I was off of it.

(Q: "How long did it usually take for that to happen?")

A week. I would stay away for a week at a time. [Eventually] I gave her to family because I was using it so much, and I was high all the time.

Dario: During most of my drug use . . . I had [two separate] apartments. I kept my wife and children, they lived in another apartment, under a different name. My wife and children were not part of my drug world.

If their partners were "straight" (non-users), household tasks such as paying rent, cleaning, fixing things and childcare were handled in the participant's absence. However, when both parents were using methamphetamine (and/or other substances), the logistics of keeping them both satisfied had to be carefully orchestrated:

Dario: If she wanted to get high I would go home, you know, every one or two weeks and I'd let her run amuck for a week. You know? I tried really hard to not let it involve the kids. I think as the addiction and the lifestyle progressed, it just eventually gave way, took away all the barriers.

Alternatively, some parents would take turns at home and, for example, go into the bathroom to get high. At times this was necessary, to keep the peace. Steve recalled that if he was high his wife would get jealous and start arguments with him, or try to give him child duty, "to break his high up."

Theme IV: Domestic Violence

Six of the participants reported being victims and/or perpetrators of domestic violence. In most cases, it seemed to be a side effect of sorts, specifically from the methamphetamine use:

Molly: I'd go from one abuser to the next. I don't know what I was looking for. The fact is, I was really passive. When I was under the influence . . . it was obvious that I wouldn't fight back. Now today, if somebody hit me, would it be one-sided? No. Nobody's gonna be mean to me.

They discussed how the drug had wreaked havoc on their moods and personalities, making them angry, argumentative and paranoid. Additionally, methamphetamine is often used as a sexual stimulant, which is one way some of the parents were introduced to it for the first time (through dating relationships). Their use progressed and increased over time, and at the height of their addictions, many claimed to have used all day, throughout the day. Warren characterized his relationship this way: "We would fight most of the day and we'd have sex most of the night." For some, the sex faded as the focus turned to the drug. Ally stated that her husband got angry with her for sleeping so much.

Two of the parents reported that they were deterred from using physical violence because they had witnessed parental domestic violence as children. They had "vowed not to do that" in front of their children. One mother claimed that she left her partner after the first time he beat her up in front of her daughter. As they described their experiences, the tone was matter-of-fact. Dario was insistent that consistency and normalcy for his children were cherished values, even in the past. However, he also described many situations that involved fights between his wife and other people. With one exception, the relationships between all the study participants and their partners were typically rocky:

Steve: I never really liked to argue in front of the kids, but my wife will argue with me anywhere. You know she'll just start screaming and hollering . . . I will call the police before I put my hands on her, but she'll beat on me, though. But I will not. No, I will not.

Ally: My child witnessed a lot of domestic violence, a whole lot. He's seen me bite [my husband] just to make him let go of my hair, while he was in my arms, my child was in my arms and I had to bite his dad to get him to let go of my hair. There was a lot of screaming.

Indeed, the children were not always bystanders. Most parents who had been involved in this kind of violence shared that their children usually tried to stop their parents from fighting by becoming either verbally or physically involved. This put them in harm's way as well:

Molly: Say he grabbed me by the throat, she might jump on his back, and the other one would try to get in the middle of it.

Marta: She would tell us both to shut up and stop fighting. She would get real upset over everything. She sensed the tension and all that between me and him, and would try and change it between both of us and tell us to talk . . . She would try to get us to sit down and play with her or something.

Domestic violence was not limited to abuse between partners. For one man, dealing methamphetamine enhanced the risk to his family. He was using and selling the drugs, as well as handling a lot of money. When asked to describe "the barriers coming down" between his methamphetamine use and his children, Dario recalled a situation in which another methamphetamine user tried to burglarize his home:

He kicks in the front door . . . punches my wife in the face. My younger son [4 years old] was on the couch. My older son [8 years old] says he was outside . . . I wound up beating the man half to death in front of the kids and my wife, who was sitting on the coffee table with her mouth bleeding and her teeth in her hands.

Theme V: The Effect on the Children

The participants readily described the physical, environmental, emotional and psychological effects of their methamphetamine use upon their children. They also discussed how this awareness had impacted their recovery, and their subsequent attempts to make amends to their children.

Physical Effects

Physically, the participants' methamphetamine use affected many of their children, literally from birth to beyond their adolescent years. For example, a few mothers used drugs during their pregnancies. Subsequently, their children tested positive and were removed from their custody. Some of the children have been removed from and returned to the home more than once. For example, CPS removed one child when he was two years old, and then again when he was eight years old. One mother admitted that one time she did not try to regain custody. A father reported fathering several children, but not knowing where many of them are today. A couple of the involved children have been molested, and/or were left in the care of inappropriate babysitters. Marta noted, "It was messed up. I gave her drugs [so she could] baby-sit my baby."

> Ally: I didn't check to see if they brushed their teeth at night . . . I didn't care if they cleaned off the table . . .

> Steve: . . . I didn't ever want to give the kids baths, you know. I mean, I didn't want to do none of that.

Environmental Effects

Maintaining safe and stable housing was a challenge, which in turn affected other aspects of the children's lives. Many parents claimed to have moved several times because they could not afford to pay rent; at times the families were homeless, either living on the streets or in a car. For some, school attendance was inconsistent. Intergenerational drug use was also commonly reported. For example, an ever-present uncle or live-in grandmother also used, and dealt methamphetamine to the parents. Two parents reported being incarcerated for drug-related crimes. As their methamphetamine use increased, the effects upon the home environment and the children intensified as well:

> Barbara: It got to the point where CPS came out. You should have seen my house. I mean . . . dishes everywhere. In my room it was disgusting . . . Oh my God, it was just one big pile of mess. You couldn't see the bed, you couldn't see nothing.

The participants reported that as they became more incapacitated by their methamphetamine use, shifts in the family systems began to occur. Some reported being divorced or separated from their partners, and subsequently having to parent alone. Informal kinship care arrangements were often made with extended family members. Additionally, their children became parentified:

> Molly: My oldest child took care of everything. I would bribe my kids into picking up the motel room, or it didn't get done . . . It would be gross . . . there'd be like moldy clothes in the closet. . . . At the end of my addiction I would be in bed and I'd still be smoking all that dope every day, but I wasn't getting out of bed . . . So they would leave for school, I would get high all day, they

would come home from school, I would still be in bed. I would not have moved.

> Natalie: My oldest knew how to work the VCR, so she would just pop in a movie, and if I was like coming down and tired, she already knew what to do, you know. . . pop in a movie, because my husband was always at work.

Psychological Effects

During the interviews, the participants shared that they were able to see some of their own behaviors in their children. They realized that they had been role models in their families, and could see indications that their children had adopted similar attitudes, as well:

> Molly: My children hate men, for the most part. And they're kind of aggressive with me because they've seen this domestic violence. And I think that when you're a kid you pick [sic], 'Well, I want to be like that.' You're not gonna be the victim, and the one being hit.

> Cheryl: He figures, okay, well my mom said it was okay, so I'll go and steal. You know, we're supposed to be their like, role models and stuff. So if I say to him okay, go rip off the store he's going to do it.

Some believed that their child's current behavioral problems are related to their time spent in foster care, or having been abused:

> Dario: Things are a bit difficult with my kids, okay, first of all, my oldest . . . was molested . . . and he in turn tried to molest [my younger son]. So for the longest time . . . [my oldest] had problems that I didn't understand. So I tried creating parenting . . . I handled it fairly well [until we moved]. Then he lit a trashcan on fire . . .

> Ally: At first you really couldn't tell, but it shows in him now before he was in foster care because he would treat me just like his dad did, he would say things to me that his dad said and not respect me . . . He's angry, very angry.

Emotional Effects

The parents speculated about the emotional damage inflicted upon the children, at times wondering out loud about what they could have done differently:

> Steve: The only thing I didn't do while I was getting high was actually spend a lot of quality time. I'm not talking the little . . . birthday thing, you know what I'm saying? I'm talking about that thing where you snuggle up and watch something on TV, or you know. . . playing a game or something, or even just sit there and talk. I never did all that while I was getting high. I never had time.

They also reported that their current treatment at the agency is confusing for the children, especially when it is paired with CPS involvement. The children ask when their parents will finish the program, and/or when they can home. The facility offers childcare while the parents are in groups, which usually enables more clients to participate. However, young children who were frequently left unattended before, or who were left for weeks at a time, had a hard time separating from the parent:

> Marta: She still has a fear of me leaving her . . . when I would tell her when I would leave I was going to the store, and not be back. So she still has that fear.

Indeed, one woman had mentioned that she still was often forgetful and had routinely showed up late when picking her children up from daycare.

Theme VI: Retrospective Ambivalence

Participants had differing opinions about whether or not they were able to handle their roles as parents while they were using methamphetamine. In the beginning of the interviews, some were quite firm that they were able to maintain a sense of order in the home. In fact, a few participants reported that at first, being high made it easier to take care of everything because the drugs gave them extra energy, and enhanced their ability to focus on their children.

> Cheryl: Before I got too far into it or whatever . . . I was level, everything was fine. I had my little stash or whatever, but I always made sure my kids were clean and they went to school, you know, made

sure they ate every day . . . When I was on it I'd cook all kinds of stuff, because you've got to be moving your hands a lot and stuff.

Steve: Actually, my awareness of the kids while I'm high is really high [sic]. Even if I'm [getting high] and heard something as far as scared or crying, if my [my wife] is fighting with the other kids, I'll stop what I'm doing.

Marta: I never had to pay for my drugs. So I would use the money that I had just for my bills, buy her clothes, diapers when she needed them . . . and whatever she needed, and the house. I would make sure she had it.

Ally: I would set times for reading . . . homework was always a must, making it to school every day was a must . . . my child never missed a day of school until the day they took her.

Other parents were unsure if their roles as parents were affected by their use. This specific question was asked near the end of the interview, after they had disclosed the general and specific impact methamphetamine use had had on their families and relationships. Many claimed to have some difficulty remembering, due to the effects of their drug use, and due to the passage of time. Some parents were ambivalent ("in a way yes, and in a way no"). Others simply responded, "I don't know." Most participants began to waver in their assertions, suggesting that there *may* have been problems in how they handled their roles. Molly was clear, however, that although she always gave her children love, it just was not enough:

I didn't think I was a bad parent. That's the really [messed up] part about all this. I was so messed up in my [sic] rational thinking and so confused about reality and what I was really doing, that I thought I was being a good parent. I was an awful mother. I made awful choices. I hurt my children.

DISCUSSION AND IMPLICATIONS

The purpose of this study was to describe how the use of methamphetamine impacts parenting. Additionally, the hope was that the findings presented would foster a better understanding of the families' experiences. To that end, both fathers and mothers were interviewed for this study. The majority of the parents had been court mandated to attend treatment, and nearly all of the families were CPS involved. Similar to other studies of the effects of drug use on parenting, the participants' self-described use of methamphetamine seemed to adversely affect the parenting role. They described isolating themselves, sleeping excessively, and at times leaving their children in unsecured environments and/or with an inappropriate caregiver. Even young children were often left unsupervised, which may have been a direct threat to their survival. Participants admitted that their attempts to be responsible were not always rational or appropriate. Instances of abandonment in public places, or "hiring" babysitters who also used drugs, for example, only served to further endanger their children. Recurrent abandonment in unsuitable environments may have affected the children's ability to trust adults to take care of them and act with their best interests at heart.

Drug use strongly impacted parents' interactions with their children. As previously stated, methamphetamine use is known to impact mood and emotional stability, which is compounded by lack of sleep. Physical effects of drug use are actually only some of the many factors affecting interpersonal interactions; drug-using parents often struggle with guilt. The tasks of handling their needs as a user as well as their children's needs can be overwhelming, leading to "minimal" parenting (Greif & Dreschsler, 1993). This is consistent with the "polar parenting" found in this study. Responding to children with flashes of anger, or alternatively, apathy, takes much less energy, forethought and self-discipline than employing a range of emotions. Instead of eliciting the children's responses, making attempts to stimulate their growth, and affirming the children's self-worth, the participants reported opposite behaviors.

Additionally, participants described the lack of appropriate parent role models, and their own histories of witnessing domestic violence between their parents. Indeed, many of the participants may have been simply applying what they have been taught through their earlier childhood experiences and social environments–and what they continue to learn in their present relationships. This finding was consistent with those of Miller, Smyth, and Mudar (1999) who found that the combination of parental and domestic violence and AOD histories resulted in higher levels of punitiveness toward their children.

The participants reported placing a great deal of energy in managing their drug use. Continuous methamphetamine use was accomplished through "careful" childproofing and the employment of alternate caregivers. Parents gave detailed descriptions of drug storage, and insisted that the substances were out of children's reach. Although it is plausible and likely that the drugs were often carefully hidden (especially because they are illegal), the gravity of the conversation did not go unnoticed. These participants may have exaggerated the truth for the benefit of the interviewer, despite the assurance of confidentiality. Factors that included their histories of losing child custody, the geographic location of the interviews, and the fact that social workers were conducting the interviews may have impacted their openness (Grant, 1996). It also may have been emotionally challenging for the participants to admit that they had left methamphetamine and/or paraphernalia within the children's reach.

Relying on the help of alternate caregivers (whether they were family or strangers) was another way these parents seemed to manage their use. Several of the parents reported having an understanding of how incapacitated they would become, and maintaining a separate life was their attempt to mediate the impact upon their children. Suchman and Luthar (2000) reported similar findings, describing the "adaptive" parenting skills drug users possess. Although the participants were at times making efforts to keep the children safe, perhaps leaving them with other people was more directly related to their not wanting to be parents; several participants described "not having the time" to respond to their children or to notice anyone else's needs outside of their own.

The participants did not report that they compensated for their drug use with their children. One mother shared that she had celebrated her child's birthday in the park when they were homeless, and there were other recollections of some holiday celebrations. Overall, however, the participants did not report daily efforts to literally make up for any of the damage they were doing to their children. Most described not realizing that the consequences of their methamphetamine use were actually bad (or at the very least, questionable), so it stands to reason that they would not attempt to offset the negatives with conscious positive behaviors.

The children were often left on their own. Older children were expected to care for younger siblings, get themselves to school, as well as maintain the home. It is expected that many of the children would exhibit behavioral problems, as Stanger et al. (1999) discussed seeing in children of drug abusers. Indeed, the participants reported that some of their children displayed separation anxiety, were outwardly angry and aggressive with them, disrespected their authority, and stole from local businesses.

Because there are so many effects of methamphetamine use, however, it becomes difficult to tease out what risk factor leads to the next one, as noted in many studies (Grant, 1996; Suchman & Luthar, 2000). The participants had many other concerns, such as lack of education or limited vocational skills, but it is difficult to address these, while they were under the influence of methamphetamine.

As their methamphetamine use increased, parents' roles, standards, and abilities to handle daily stress changed over time. Hardesty and Black (1999) reported that the women in their study believed that they had maintained decent standards of childrearing. Even if the mothers struggled with drug use, their ability to mother well was a source of pride that served to enhance their self-esteem. This may be one reason many participants in this study were initially unwilling to fathom the idea that their parenting had been impacted by their methamphetamine use. It may have been difficult for some of the parents to admit to compromising the health and safety of their children due to the resulting guilt and damage to their own self-images as fathers or mothers.

Interestingly, several participants in this study were insistent that no matter what, their children were routinely fed, read to, clothed, and that they went to school each day. These are obviously only fractions of parental responsibility, but if some participants were better able to handle the parenting role over longer periods of time, it may have been due to certain personality traits that buffer the impact of their drug use on their children.

The participants were all willing to disclose details regarding the inevitable deterioration of their parenting standards. They gave a fairly comprehensive picture of their homes and abilities prior to CPS involvement: filthy environments, child neglect, an inability to pay bills (including rent), nonexistent motivation, and for some, homelessness. It was, however, difficult for the participants to actually delineate when their use became "really" damaging to their children and they spent minimal time discussing their parenting capabilities while under the influence of methamphetamine. The overwhelming response was that their lives became unmanageable because they were literally incapacitated. Questions regarding their handling of stress were moot; they "weren't handling anything" at that point. In reviewing the results presented, there is no question that, throughout their use and to the end, their methamphetamine use greatly impacted their abilities to parent and respond to their children.

Participants shared common but detrimental parenting behaviors, fundamental beliefs and subsequent consequences that have been magnified and prolonged due to methamphetamine use. Families certainly may differ in their experiences. Results of this study, however, do indicate a need for a shift from individual drug treatment to a comprehensive family recovery plan. Mandated treatment for methamphetamine use could include family therapy in addition to individual treatment, as well as marital counseling, if appropriate. Treatment also needs to include parenting classes and on-site childcare, so that clients would have many opportunities to ask questions and practice new skills. Volunteer time in the childcare center could be an important part of the treatment plan.

There is also a clear need to collaborate with outside agencies that include but extend beyond drug treatment counselors, CPS workers, and police officers. Assessment tools should include questions exploring the possibility of parental methamphetamine abuse.

School social workers could provide information about the impact of methamphetamine use on family systems to teachers and support staff by means of in-services and informal conversation. Even if children of methamphetamine abusers are going to school, the struggle to feel safe, loved, and a sense of belonging in their own homes could be impairing their abilities to be successful in school.

Because methamphetamine abusers may have long histories of use while parenting, outreach is important. Communities need to be continually informed of the hazards of methamphetamine abuse–as well as the available treatment and support programs. Providing treatment to clients with younger children may serve to avert future damage. It might also enhance a family's ability to be successful in treatment because the negative patterns of behavior would not be as firmly ingrained.

LIMITATIONS

The main limitation of this study was its small sample size, and the fact that the participants were mandated to attend treatment. Additionally, all of the participants were self-selected and came from one agency, which may have biased the findings. Also, many of the participants had been in treatment for only a few months; it would be helpful to have obtained interviews from those in varied stages of treatment and recovery. For example, people who have been in drug treatment for longer period of time may have more insight about their parenting. They may also have more time to practice incorporating new behaviors into their daily lifestyles, and thus may feel more secure in discussing their experiences because they are no longer breaking the law. Participants with limited recovery are more likely to relapse, or to be suffering the residual effects of drug use and exposure (Grant, 1996). This may affect their abilities to recall and report accurate information. Mandated clients, in particular, may also choose to withhold or alter information if they think disclosure will negatively impact their cases in court or with CPS. They may in fact be less truthful, especially due to the interviewer's status as a mandated reporter. For example, although the Certificate of Confidentiality protects those involved against the disclosure of past instances of abuse and/or neglect of minors and the elderly, the interviewer was legally bound to report current instances of abuse and/or neglect, which was made known to all of the participants.

In summary, due to the limited sample pool and small sample size, no generalizations from this study can be made. However, knowledge gained regarding this topic may serve to guide future, larger studies of methamphetamine-using parents. Future research needs to examine the parental patterns found in this study in larger samples. Studies also need to examine the relationships between the parental patterns and their children's behaviors.

REFERENCES

Anglin, M.D., Burke, C., Perrochet, B., Stamper, E., & Dawud-Noursi, S. (2000). History of the methamphetamine problem. *Journal of Psychoactive Drugs, 32* (2), 137-141.

Beebe, D., & Walley, E. (1995). Smokable methamphetamine ('ice'): An old drug in a different form. *American Family Physician, 51* (2), 449-453.

Brecht, M.-L., O'Brien, A., von Mayerhauser, C., & Anglin, M. D. (2004). Methamphetamine use behaviors and gender differences. *Addictive Behaviors, 29*, 89-106.

Brown, J. (2001). *An agency assessment: ParentCare.* Unpublished manuscript.

Community Epidemiology Work Group. (2000). *Epidemiology trends in drug abuse.* Rockville, MD: National Institute of Drug Abuse.

Cohen, J. B., Dickow, A., Horner, K., Zweben, J. E., Balabis, J., Vandersloot, D., & Reiber C. (2003). Abuse and violence history of men and women in treatment for methamphetamine dependence. *American Journal on Addictions, 12* (5), 377-385.

Cretzmeyer, M., Sarrazin, M. V., Huber, D. L., Block, R. I., & Hall, J. A. (2003). Treatment of methamphetamine abuse: Research findings and clinical directions. *Journal of Substance Abuse Treatment, 24*, 267-277.

Ells, M., Sturgis, B., & Wright, G. (2002). Behind the drug: The child victims of meth labs. *American Prosecutors Research Institute, 15* (2), 1-7. Available at *http://www.ndaa-apri.org/pubications/newletters.* Accessed September 2, 2003.

Gibson, D.R., Leamon, M.H., & Flynn, N. (2002). Epidemiology and public health consequences of methamphetamine use in California's Central valley. *Journal of Psychoactive Drugs, 34* (3), 313-318.

Gorman, E. M., Clark, C. W., Nelson, K. R., Applegate, T., Amato, E., & Scrol, A. (2003). A community social work study of methamphetamine use among women: Implications for social work practice, education, and research. *Journal of Social Work Practice in the Addictions, 3* (3), 41-62.

Grant, D. (1996). Generalizability of findings of exploratory practice-based research on polydrug-addicted mothers. *Research on Social Work Practice, 6* (3), 292-308.

Greif, G., & Drechsler, M. (1993). Common issues for parents in a methadone mainte- nance group. *Journal of Substance Abuse Treatment, 10,* 339-343.

Hardesty, M., & Black, T. (1999). Mothering through addiction: A survival strategy among Puerto Rican addicts. *Qualitative Health Research, 9* (5), 602-619.

Harrington, D., Dubowitz, H., Black, M., & Binder, A. (1995). Maternal substance use and neglectful parenting: Relations with children's development. *Journal of Clini- cal Child Psychology, 24* (3), 258-263.

Hogan, D. (1998). Annotation: The psychological development and welfare of chil- dren of opiate and cocaine users: Review and research needs. *Journal of Child Psy- chology & Psychiatry, 39* (5), 609-620.

Hohman, M., Oliver, R., & Wright, W. (2004). Methamphetamine abuse, manufacture, and the child welfare response. *Social Work, 49* (3), 373-382.

Hohman, M., Shillington, A., & Clapp, J. (2002). *A comparison of methamphetamine- using and cocaine-using women in the public treatment system.* Unpublished manu- script.

Irvine, G.D., & Chin, L. (1997). The environmental impact and adverse health effects of the clandestine manufacture of methamphetamine. *Substance Use and Misuse, 32* (12 & 13), 1811-1812.

Mayes, L. (1995). Substance abuse and parenting. In M.H. Bornstein (Ed.), *Handbook of parenting* (pp. 101-125). Mahwah, NJ: Lawrence Erlbaum.

Miles, M.B., & Huberman, A.M. (Eds.). (1994). *Qualitative data analysis: An ex- panded sourcebook* (2nd ed.). Thousand Oaks, CA: Sage.

Miller, B., Smyth, N., & Mudar, P. (1999). Mothers' alcohol and other drug problems and their punitiveness toward their children. *Journal of Studies on Alcohol, 60,* 632-642.

Murray, J. B. (1998). Psychophysiological aspects of amphetamine-methamphetamine abuse. *The Journal of Psychology, 132* (2), 227-237.

National Institute of Justice (1999). *ADAM: 1998 annual report on adult and juvenile arrestees.* Washington, DC: U.S. Department of Justice, (NIJ Publication NCJ 175660).

Nurco, D., Blatchley, R., Hanlon, T., O'Grady, K., & McCarren, M. (1998). The family experiences of narcotic addicts and their subsequent parenting practices. *American Journal of Drug and Alcohol Abuse. 24* (1), 37-59.

Padgett, D. K. (1998). *Qualitative methods in social work: Challenges and rewards.* Thousand Oaks, CA: Sage.

Rawson, R. A. (1999). *Treatment for stimulant use disorders.* TIP Series #33. Rockville, MD: U.S. Department of Health and Human Services.

Reiber, C., Galloway, G., Cohen, J., Hsu, J. C., & Lord, R. H. (2000). A descriptive analysis of participant characteristics and patterns of substance use in the CSAT methamphetamine treatment project: The first six months. *Journal of Pyschoactive Drugs, 32* (2), 157-164.

Stalcup, A. (April, 2000). *Methamphetamine use and treatment.* Paper presented at the California Association of Alcohol and Drug Educators, San Diego.

Stanger, C., Higgins, S., Bickel, W., Elk, R., Grabowski, J., Schmitz, J., Amass, L., Kirby, K., & Seracini, A. (1999). Behavioral and emotional problems among children of cocaine- and opiate-dependent parents. *Journal of the American Academy of Child and Adolescent Psychiatry. 38* (4), 421-427.

Substance Abuse and Mental Health Services Administration [SAMHSA] (2001). *Amphetamine treatment admissions increase: 1992-1999.* Office of Applied Studies, Substance Abuse and Mental Health Services Administration, TEDS 4.16.01. Available at *http://www.samhsa.gov/oas/facts/Speed.pdf.* Accessed September 2, 2003.

Suchman, N., & Luthar, S. (2000). Maternal addiction, child maladjustment and sociodemographic risks: Implications for parenting behaviors. *Addiction, 95* (9), 1417-1429.

Tutty, L. M., Rothery, M. A., & Grinnell, R. M. (1996). *Qualitative research for social workers.* Boston: Allyn and Bacon.

Wermuth, L. (2000). Methamphetamine use: Hazards and social influences. *Drug Education, 30* (4), 423-433.

The Child in the Family
of a Drug-Using Father:
Attachment Styles
and Family Characteristics

Ricky Finzi-Dottan
Orna Cohen
Dorota Iwaniec
Yaffa Sapir
Abraham Weizman

SUMMARY. The study examined the impact of family characteristics and parental attachment styles on the children of drug-using (DU) fathers in fifty-six families (n = 168) in Israel. Of the DU fathers, 60.7%

Ricky Finzi-Dottan, PhD, is Senior Lecturer, Bar Ilan University, School of Social Work, Ramat Gan, Israel 52900 (E-mail: rikifinz@mail.biu.ac.il). Orna Cohen, PhD, is faculty member, Bob Shappell School of Social Work, Tel Aviv University, Ramat-Aviv, Israel 69978 (E-mail: oracoh@post.tau.ac.il). Dorota Iwaniec, PhD, is Director, Institute of Child Care Research, Queen's University, Belfast, 7 Lennoxvale, Belfast BT9 5BY, Northern Ireland (E-mail: D.iwaniec@Queens-Belfast.ac.uk). Yaffa Sapir, PhD, is Program Planner, Central School for Social Welfare Workers, Ministry of Labor and Social Affairs, Tel Aviv, Israel (E-mail: sapiry@netvision.net.il). Abraham Weizman, MD, is Professor of Psychiatry, Sackle Faculty of Medicine, Tel Aviv University, and Head of the Research Department, Geha Mental Health Center, Petach-Tiqva, Israel.

[Haworth co-indexing entry note]: "The Child in the Family of a Drug-Using Father: Attachment Styles and Family Characteristics." Finzi-Dottan, Ricky et al. Co-published simultaneously in *Journal of Social Work Practice in the Addictions* (The Haworth Press, Inc.) Vol. 6, No. 1/2, 2006, pp. 89-111; and: *Impact of Substance Abuse on Children and Families: Research and Practice Implications* (ed: Shulamith Lala Ashenberg Straussner, and Christine Huff Fewell) The Haworth Press, Inc., 2006, pp. 89-111. Single or multiple copies of this article are available for a fee from The Haworth Document Delivery Service [1-800-HAWORTH, 9:00 a.m. - 5:00 p.m. (EST). E-mail address: docdelivery@haworthpress.com].

Available online at http://www.haworthpress.com/web/JSWPA
doi:10.1300/J160v06n01_05

were characterized by avoidant attachment style. Among the non-DU mothers, 53.6% were characterized by secure attachment style, 42.9% by avoidant style, and 3.6% by anxious/ambivalent style. Surprisingly, family cohesion and adaptability scores were similar to the Israeli norm, perhaps because the DUs had completed detoxification treatment and participated in rehabilitation programs. Of the children, 61.8% were characterized by secure attachment style, 21.8% by avoidant style, and 16.4% by anxious/ambivalent style. Stepwise regression to predict children's attachment styles revealed that maternal security of attachment and paternal anxious/ambivalent style predict similar attachment styles among the children. The important combined effects of spousal attachment styles on the children are discussed. *[Article copies available for a fee from The Haworth Document Delivery Service: 1-800-HAWORTH. E-mail address: <docdelivery@haworthpress.com> Website: <http://www.Haworth Press.com> © 2006 by The Haworth Press, Inc. All rights reserved.]*

KEYWORDS. Children of drug-using fathers, family cohesion and adaptability, attachment styles, parental impact

INTRODUCTION

Drug addiction becomes a "career" that encompasses all aspects of addicts' lives and of that of their families. The needs and well-being of other family members become secondary to the addict's needs, around whom the entire family life revolves. The addiction affects family relations, spousal life style, and especially the lives of the children.

A substantial body of literature has revealed that parental drug abuse causes a variety of problems in family dynamics. Clinical studies have emphasized dysfunctional internal and external boundaries (Isaacson, 1991; MacKensen & Cottone, 1992), poor communication skills, low expressiveness, and high rate of family conflict (Crnkovic & DelCampo, 1998; Hogan, 1998; Isaacson, 1991); chaotic or rigid interaction patterns (Dore, Kauffman, & Nelson-Zlupko, 1996; National Center on Child Abuse and Neglect (NCCAN), 1994); and role distortion and role reversal (Bekir, McLellan, Childress, & Gariti, 1993; Cook, 1991; Dore, Kauffman, & Nelson-Zlupko, 1996). Low levels of family competence and adverse family environment have also been noted (Crnkovic & DelCampo, 1998; Sheridan, 1995). Empirical studies have found dysfunctional family relations (Lavee & Altus, 2001), low levels of family cohesion and adaptability, and co-dependant relations between drug-user (DU) husbands and their non-DU wives (Teichman & Basha, 1996).

Children whose parents misuse drugs are at high risk for neglect and abuse (Dore, 1995; Famularo, Kinscherff, & Fenton, 1992; Sheridan, 1995; Wilens, Biderman, Kiely, Bredin, & Spencer, 1995; Wolock & Magura, 1996) and a chaotic child-rearing environment (Garbarino & Vondra, 1987). These children may be subject to developmental impairments and show behavioral problems (Clark, Moss, Kirisci, Mezzich, Miles, & Ott, 1997; Hogan, 1998; NCCAN, 1994; Rivinus, Levoy, Matzko, & Seifer, 1992; Wilens et al., 1995).

Drug abusing parents frequently model impulsivity and an inability to delay gratification or cope with frustration (Dore et al., 1996; Gabel & Schindledecker, 1992; Scherling, 1994). Drug addicts are often moody, difficult to comprehend, and may cause constant anxiety to the child who must anticipate when the parent is likely to become violent or self-destructive. Furthermore, witnessing a parent losing control over his/her physical or cognitive functioning is frightening and shameful for the child (Dore et al., 1996). Learning from an early age to keep the family secret may cause feelings of isolation and fear of peer rejection (Dore et al., 1996). The chaotic environment, often combined with unrealistic parental expectations and perceptions regarding the child's needs, may drive children to assume a parental role, including taking care of themselves and their siblings, or parenting their parents (Bekir et al., 1993; Cook, 1991). The children learn to repress their wishes, feelings (especially anger), and needs, and become expert readers of the emotional state of their addicted parent (Crnkovic & DelCampo, 1998; Dore et al., 1996). While clinical descriptions shed light on various aspects of the reality of children exposed to familial drug-addiction, they lack a conceptual framework that can be studied empirically.

Attachment theory has been offered as one way of explaining the relation between family experiences of children and their social and emotional development (Ainsworth, 1989; Bowlby, 1973, 1977), and there is a large literature on this topic. Surprisingly, however, information about attachment in DU families and the effects on children's development is sparse. Most of the existing studies focus on parenting by DU mothers (Hogan, 1998) rather than fathers. Therefore, this study focused on families with a DU father and the impact of parental attachment styles on the children.

ATTACHMENT THEORY AND THE FAMILY

Attachment is the core bond influencing the ways families provide care and protection over the life cycle (Ainsworth, 1989; Byng-Hall, 1999). Bowlby (1973, 1977) theorized that the nature and quality of attachment relationships are largely determined by a "secure base" of emotional availability and responsiveness of the caregiver to the child's needs. According to Bowlby (1988), the development of "internal working models,"–the internalized representations of the self and others–produces in infants a repertoire of behavioral skills and affective responses that are reflected, reinforced, and modified in their future interactions (Bretherton, Ridgeway, & Cassidy, 1990).

Ainsworth, Blehar, Waters, and Wall (1978) operationalized attachment theory. Based on structured laboratory observations of infants and their caregivers, they proposed a taxonomy of three main categories of attachment styles: secure, avoidant, and anxious/ambivalent. These attachment patterns affect functioning in areas such as social skills, functional/dysfunctional relationships, affect regulation, and coping with stressful situations over the life-span (Ainsworth, 1989). Thus, children with a secure attachment style develop better problem solving abilities and show more co-operation and empathy in interpersonal relationships, more ego resiliency, and better cognitive performance. Children characterized by an anxious/ambivalent style tend to be dependent, to have anxiety problems, and to be easily irritated because of impairments in their emotional regulation. Finally, children characterized by an avoidant attachment style tend to demonstrate hostility, aggressive behavior, emotional insulation, and lack of empathy (Weinfield, Sroufe, Egeland, & Carlson 1999).

In the last two decades scholarly attention has extended to adult attachment styles (Simpson & Rholes, 1998). The pioneers in this field, Hazan and Shaver (1987), contend that attachment theory can describe how adults with different attachment styles think, feel, and behave in close relationships. Hazan and Shaver (1994) have defined adult individuals with a secure style as possessing confidence in the accessibility of significant others in times of need and demonstrating comfort with closeness and interdependence. The adult with an avoidant style is defined by insecurity about the responses of others and by a desire for emotional distance. The individual with an anxious/ambivalent style, while also defined by insecurity about responses of others has at the same time a strong desire for intimacy and a fear of rejection.

Studies indicate that attachment style is related to the quality of marital relations (Collins & Read, 1990; Feeney, 1996; Mikulincer & Florian, 1999), and to family and parental behavior toward children (Berlin & Cassidy, 1999; Cohen, Cowan, Cowan, & Pearson, 1992; George & Solomon, 1999; Marvin & Stewart, 1990). Mikulincer and Florian (1999) indicated that adults with a secure attachment reported relatively high levels of family cohesion (namely, emotional bonding) and adaptability (the ability of a family to change its power structure, roles, and relationship rules in response to situational and developmental stress). Individuals with an anxious-ambivalent style reported high levels of family cohesion, but low levels of adaptability; those with an avoidant style reported relatively low levels of both family adaptability and cohesion.

The present study examined Israeli families with DU husbands and their non-DU wives after the husband had completed detoxification from drugs. The aim of the study was twofold: (1) to shed light on the parents' personal characteristics (attachment style) and their view of their family characteristics (cohesion and adaptability) that might facilitate the husband's rehabilitation; and (2) to examine the impact of living in the shade of paternal addiction on the attachment style of their children.

METHOD

Participants

The study population consisted of 168 subjects belonging to 56 families: 56 DU husbands in the first-stages of recovery from addiction after detoxification; their wives (N = 56) who were not DUs; and the youngest child in the family (N = 56). The participating DUs were undergoing rehabilitation in outpatient units for the treatment of DUs in Israel after completing the detoxification program.

The mean age of the husbands was 38.9 years (SD = 5.15). The majority (54.5%) began to use drugs before the age of 15; 34.5% before the age of 20; and 10.9% after the age of 21. Most (52.9%) used heroin; 27.5% used a combination of drugs; and the others used heroin and cocaine. A majority of the men underwent detoxification more than once: 57.4% had been through 2-5 detoxification treatments, and 33.3% underwent more than 6 treatments.

The mean age of the wives was 35.61 years (SD = 5.68). The couples had been married for a long time: 42.9% had been married for over 16 years, the rest for at least 6 years. Most of them had 3 to 4 children. Of the 56 children studied, 25 (44.7%) were boys and 31 (55.3%) girls. The children were between 7-14 years old, with a mean age of 10.86 (SD = 2.55). More than two-thirds of the participants defined their socioeconomic status as middle class, and one-third as lower.

The participants were recruited on a voluntary basis by social workers in outpatient units for the treatment of drug abusers in Israel; all had been referred to the units within the previous two months. DU husbands and their wives gave informed consent after the objectives of the study were explained to them. The aims of the research were explained to the children and the option to refuse to answer questions or to continue with the study were discussed.

Instruments

Two instruments were administered to the adults. Attachment was measured using the *Adult Attachment Style Classification Questionnaire* (Mikulincer, Florian, & Tolmacz, 1990). This is the Hebrew version of Hazan and Shaver's (1987) instrument. It includes three brief statements designed as direct adult analogue of Ainsworth's classification of attachment types in infancy. Each statement contains a description of feelings and attitudes that characterize one of the three attachment styles. In the Hebrew version, Mikulincer, Florian, and Tolmacz (1990) broke down these three statements and composed a continuous measure consisting of 15 sentences, five for each attachment style, based on Likert-type scales ranging from 1 (strongly disagree) to 7 (strongly agree). Cronbach's alpha for each of the attachment styles yielded a high internal consistency (secure style: $\alpha = .85$; anxious/ambivalent style: $\alpha = .79$; avoidant style: $\alpha = .83$). The Hebrew instrument was validated in several studies (e.g., Mikulincer, 1997).

The second instrument administered to adults was *FACES III* (Olson, 1986; translated into Hebrew by Teichman & Navon, 1990). This is a self-report questionnaire designed to measure family cohesion and adaptability. It consists of two subscales, Cohesion and Adaptability, each containing 10 items. Subjects rated the extent to which each item reflected their current perceptions of their family on a 5-point Likert scale, ranging from 1 (almost never) to 5 (almost always). Previous studies reported high internal consistency coefficients and high test-retest reliability for each of the subscales, as well as low correlations with measures of social desirability (Olson, 1986; Teichman & Navon, 1990).

Children's attachment was measured by the *Children's Attachment Style Classification Questionnaire* (Finzi, Har-Even, Weizman, Tyano, & Shnit, 1996; Finzi, Cohen, & Ram, 2000). This questionnaire is an adaptation for children of the Adult Attachment Style Classification Questionnaire (described above). The questionnaire contains 15 items divided into three attachment factors: secure (e.g., "I make friends with other children easily"), anxious/ambivalent (e.g., "I sometimes feel that others don't want to be good friends with me as much as I do with them"), and avoidant (e.g., "It's hard for me to really trust others, even if they're good friends of mine"). The children were asked to read each item and to rate the extent to which the item described them on a 5-point scale, with scores ranging from 1 (not at all) to 5 (very much). The psychometric properties and concurrent validity of the questionnaire were evaluated in 232 elementary school children, half boys and half girls (mean age 9.2, SD = 2.1 years). A principal component factor analysis with varimax rotation yielded three factors (eigenvalues > 1) with items loading in the range of .40-.55. Cronbach's alpha for each of the attachment styles yielded a reasonable internal consistency (α = .69-.81). The test-retest stability after two weeks was in the high range (r = .87-.95). Concurrent validity was evaluated by Pearson's correlation with children's scores on the Trait Anxiety Inventory (Spielberger, Edwards, Lushene, Montuori, & Platzek, 1973), Child Depression Inventory (Kovacs, 1992), and Child Suicidal Potential Scales (which also assesses levels of aggressiveness) (Pfeffer, Lipkins, Plutchik, & Mizruchi, 1988). Low depression, anxiety, and aggression levels characterized children with a secure style. High depression and anxiety levels characterized children with an avoidant or anxious/ambivalent style, and high aggression level characterized children with an avoidant style. The distribution of attachment styles among latency age children was similar to that found in previous studies of infants, toddlers, and adults (Hazan & Shaver, 1987).

RESULTS

Family Dimensions: Cohesion and Adaptability

The husbands and their wives completed the FACES III questionnaire separately. MANOVA analysis comparing the responses of husbands and wives did not reveal significant differences between them [$F(2,53) = 1.84$; $p > 0.05$]. For comparison with the general population, we used the Teichman and Navon (1990) norm for family cohesion and adaptability, which was established in a research study using a sample of 400 Israelis (aged 18 to 54 years). Analysis of variance revealed no significant differences. Table 1 presents the means and standard deviations of the cohesion and adaptability scores of DU husbands and their wives in comparison to Israeli norm.

Because no significant differences were found in the perception of family dimensions (cohesion and adaptability) between the DU fathers and their wives, we used a mean score in the following sections to reflect the scores of both.

Attachment Styles

The drug users and their wives were classified into one of three attachment styles according to their attachment factor scores. MANOVA analysis yielded significant differences in attachment styles between DUs and their wives ($F(3,53) = 4.76$; $p < .01$). The husbands were less secure than their wives (DU M = 4.15, SD = 1.39 vs. wives M = 4.55, SD = 1.32), more avoidant (DU M = 4.67, SD = 1.14 vs. wives M = 4.17, SD = 1.18), and more anxious/ambivalent (DU M = 3.70, SD = 1.34 vs. wives M = 3.03, SD = 1.29).

Among DU men, the majority, 60.7% (N = 34), were classified as avoidant, 26.8% (N = 15) as secure, and 12.5% (N = 7) as anxious/ambivalent. Of the wives, 53.6% (N = 30) were classified as secure, 42.9% (N = 24) as avoidant, and 3.6% (N = 2) as anxious/ambivalent. Chi-

TABLE 1. Family Cohesion and Adaptability: DUs and Their Wives vs. the Israeli Norm

	Cohesiveness		Adaptability	
	Mean	SD	Mean	SD
Drug users (n = 56)	37.48	7.86	29.35	6.02
Wives (n = 56)	36.58	6.97	30.10	6.94
Norm (n = 400)	37.48	6.35	28.62	5.54
F (1,54) Wives	0.01		0.90	
DU Husbands	0.81		3.40	

square analysis revealed significant differences between DUs and their wives ($\chi^2 = 8.72$; df = 2; p < .05).

These results were compared with a non-clinical Israeli population (Mikulincer, 1995). Chi-square analysis revealed significant differences between the DUs and the non-clinical population ($\chi^2 = 41.24$; df = 2; p < 0.001) and between the wives of DUs and their corresponding controls ($\chi^2 = 9.54$; df = 2; p < 0.01). DUs were characterized by less secure style than the Israeli norm (26.8 % vs. 63%, respectively), more avoidant (60.7% vs. 24%), and similar in the anxious/ambivalent style (12.5% vs. 13%). The wives of DUs were characterized by less anxious/ambivalent style (3.6 % vs. 13%), more avoidant style (42.9% vs. 24%), and similar in the secure style (53.6% vs. 63%) compared to wives of non-DUs.

The combination of spousal attachment styles indicated that: 34% of the couples showed combined secure and avoidant attachment styles, in 31% of the couples both spouses were classified as avoidant, in 13% of the couples both spouses were classified as secure, in 10% one spouse was classified as secure and the other as anxious/ambivalent, in 7% as avoidant and anxious/ambivalent and in 5% of the couples both spouses were classified as anxious/ambivalent (see Table 2).

Among the children, 61.8% (N = 35) were classified as secure, 21.8% (N = 12) as avoidant, and 16.4% (N = 9) as anxious/ambivalent. The mean of the secure factor was 3.77 (SD = .58), of the avoidant factor M = 3.08 (SD = .65), and of the anxious/ambivalent factor M = 2.76 (SD = .89). Analysis of variance yielded no significant differences between gender ($F(3,51) = .68$; p > .05) or age ($F (2,47) = .52$; p > .05) in the three attachment factors.

Family Cohesion and Adaptability, Parental Attachment Styles, and Children's Attachment Styles

First, we examined the associations between the DUs and their wives' attachment styles and family cohesion and adaptability. Pearson's cor-

TABLE 2. Distribution of the Couples' Attachment Styles Combinations

	Secure	Avoidant	Anxious/ambivalent
Secure	13%	34%	10%
Avoidant		31%	7%
Anxious/ambivalent			5%

relation yielded significant positive correlations between family cohesion and the secure style in DUs and their wives (.34 and .26), and significant negative correlations with the anxious/ambivalent style in DUs and their wives (.28 and .43). A significant positive correlation was found in family adaptability of DUs with secure attachment style (.23).

Associations between the children's attachment styles and family dimensions (cohesion and adaptability) on the one hand, and parental attachment styles on the other, were examined by Pearson correlation. As can be seen in Table 3, significant positive correlations were found between children with secure attachment style, maternal secure and paternal avoidant style, and family cohesion and adaptability; and a significant negative correlation was found between children with secure attachment style and maternal insecure styles (anxious/ambivalent and avoidant). Children with anxious/ambivalent style showed significant negative correlations with family dimensions, and significant positive correlations with anxious/ambivalent paternal style. Finally, children with avoidant style had significant negative correlation with anxious/ambivalent paternal style.

Predicting Children's Attachment Styles

A stepwise hierarchic regression was calculated to predict the children's attachment styles by family dimensions (cohesion and adaptabil-

TABLE 3. Pearson's Correlation Between Children's Attachment Styles, Family Cohesion and Adaptability, and Parents' Attachment Styles

Children / Parents	Secure	Anxious/Ambivalent	Avoidant
Family Cohesion	.19*	−.26*	−.01
Family Adaptability	.23*	−.21*	.01
DU Secure	.12	−.08	.07
Mo. Secure	.27*	−.07	−.50
DU Anx.	−.01	.27*	−.25*
Mo. Anx.	−.20*	.06	−.16
DU Av.	.22*	−.04	.05
Mo. Av.	−.22*	.12	−.05

*p < .05
Note: DU = Drug-user father; Mo = mother; S = Secure attachment style; Anx = Anxious/ambivalent attachment style; Av = Avoidant attachment style.

ity) and parental attachment styles. Table 4 presents the predictors for children's secure style and Table 5 the predictors of children's anxious/ambivalent attachment styles. Family and parental variables were not found to contribute to children's avoidant style. In these two regressions (Tables 4 and 5) the family dimensions did not contribute to the prediction, probably because of the high correlation with parental attachment styles.

The hierarchic regressions predicting children's secure attachment style reflected in Table 4 show that in the first step significant contributors were maternal secure attachment style, maternal avoidant attachment style (negative contribution), and DU fathers' avoidant attachment style, explaining 18% of the variance; in the second step, the interaction of maternal secure with avoidant style explained an additional 6% of the variance.

To examine the interaction between maternal secure attachment style and avoidant style the mothers' scores for both attachment styles were divided according to the medians and averages were calculated for each of the four subgroups. This analysis revealed that children of mothers who scored high in the avoidant and low in the secure style were less secure than children whose mothers' attachment style scores were different. Hierarchic regressions for predicting children's anxious/ ambivalent attach-

TABLE 4. Stepwise Regression Predicting Children's Secure Style by Family Dimensions and Parental Attachment Styles

Predictors	β	B	SEB	ΔR^2
Step 1				.18*
Mo S	.30**	.16	.06	
Mo Av	−.23*	−.13	.07	
DU Av	.22*	.13	.08	
Step 2				.06**
Mo S	.27**	.14	.06	
Mo Av	−.23*	−.13	.07	
Du Av	.19	.11	.08	
Mo S × Mo Av	.23*	.17	.09	

*p < .05, **p < .01
Note: DU = Drug-user father; Mo = mother; S = Secure attachment style; Anx = Anxious/ambivalent attachment style; Av = Avoidant attachment style.

TABLE 5. Stepwise Regression Predicting Children's Anxious/Ambivalent Attachment Style by Family Dimensions and Parental Attachment Styles

Predictors	β	B	SEB	ΔR^2
Step 1				.07*
DU Anx	.27**	.18	.09	
Step 2				.08*
DU Anx	.33*	.22	.09	
DU S × DU Av	−.29**	−.22	.10	

*p < .05, **p < .01
Note: DU = Drug-user father; S = Secure attachment style; Anx = Anxious/ambivalent attachment style; Av = Avoidant attachment style.

ment style (Table 5) explained 7% of the variance in the first step looking at paternal anxious/ambivalent style, while in the second step, the interaction of paternal secure and avoidant style explained further 8% of the variance.

To examine the interaction between paternal secure attachment style and the avoidant style, the fathers' scores for the secure and avoidant attachment styles were divided according to the medians and averages were calculated for each of the four subgroups. This analysis revealed that children of fathers who scored high in the avoidant and low in the secure style were less anxious/ambivalent than children whose fathers' attachment style scores were different.

DISCUSSION

This study examined attachment styles and family cohesion and adaptability in 168 members of families with DU fathers and non-DU mothers in which the fathers completed detoxification and were now attending an outpatient treatment program.

The findings of this study concerning family dimensions were surprising because no difference was found between the Israeli norm and the way DU husbands and their wives perceived their family adaptability and cohesion. These results are inconsistent with previous descriptions of families affected by drug addiction, which were found to be characterized by disengagement (Friedman, Utada, & Morrissey, 1987), dysfunctional boundaries, ambiguous communication, chaotic, or rigid interaction, and high rate of family conflicts (Crnkovic & DelCampo, 1998; Sheridan, 1995), all of which affect cohesion and adaptability (Makensen & Cottone, 1992). Our results may be attributed to the involvement of both spouses in the family-based rehabilitation program, which may have contributed to their belief that this time, together, they would overcome the drug use. This assumption is supported by a previous study by Teichman and Basha (1996), which reported scores similar to the Israeli norm as the treatment progressed. These perceptions, apparent during later stages in the rehabilitation process, may promote recovery by continued mutual spousal support (Kang, Kleinman, Todd, & Kemp, 1991).

Attachement Styles of DU Husbands and Their Wives

One of the personal resources that affects the ability to cope with stressful experiences is attachment style (Diehl, Elnick, Bourbeau, & Labouvie-Vief, 1998; Meyers, 1998). Attachment models may function as internalized mental structures by which individuals organize experience and handle distress. A secure attachment style is an inner resource that may help a person to appraise stressful experiences positively, to constructively cope with psychological distress and to improve personal well-being and adjustment. In contrast, insecure attachment style, either avoidant or anxious/ambivalent, can be viewed as a potential risk factor that in times of stress may detract from the individual's resilience, leading to poor coping and to maladjustment (Mikulincer & Florian, 1999). Our findings indicated that most of the DUs were characterized by avoidant attachment style while their wives' attachment style distribution was significantly different, with approximately half of them characterized by secure style. The attachment style variable shed light on the DUs' personal ability to cope with the rehabilitation process and on their wives' resources for coping with family strain and promoting the recovery of their husbands (Hofler & Kooyman, 1996). It also shed light on parental ability to be attentive and sensitive to children's distress caused by the paternal addiction (Plasse, 1995).

Research dealing with the attachment styles of DUs is scarce and research investigating the attachment styles of their spouses is even more rare. From existing research it is possible to infer that people with a secure attachment style are able to balance intimacy and autonomy, separateness and connectedness (Belsky & Cassidy, 1994; Collins & Read, 1990; Feeney, 1996). They trust others and are able to share their feelings and ask for help (Hazan & Shaver, 1994); their communication skills tend to be good (Senchak & Leonard, 1992); they can integrate conflicting emotions, regulate negative emotions, solve conflicts jointly and constructively (Pistole, 1989; Kobak & Hazan, 1991), and employ more constructive coping strategies in crises (Birnbaum, Orr, Mikulincer, & Florian, 1997). These features may enable the DU and his wife to cope more efficiently with the recovery process.

Research about individuals with the two insecure styles portrays them as less well equipped to cope with this difficult period. Persons with an avoidant attachment style tend to lack empathy and to undervalue the importance of close relationships. They distance themselves from the needs of others and avoid intimate relationships, which they find threatening (Belsky & Cassidy, 1994; Shaver & Hazan, 1994). Although they need to perceive and present themselves as highly self-reliant, they are extremely sensitive to rejection (Bartholomew, 1997; Belsky & Cassidy, 1994; Hazan & Shaver, 1994), deny feelings of distress and insecurity (Mikulincer & Nachson, 1991), and thus often harbor considerable and easily triggered rage (Rusbult, Verette, Whitney, Solvik, & Lipkus, 1991; Sharpsteen & Kirkpatrick, 1997). They are described as rigid, with a narrow response repertoire and poor conflict solving skills (Kobak & Hazan, 1991; Pistole, 1989).

Persons with an anxious/ambivalent attachment style tend to exaggerate the importance of proximity, intimacy, involvement, and connectedness almost to the point of interpersonal fusion. They tend to suffer from anxiety and self-doubt, and to be obsessive or preoccupied with emotional security in their relationships (Belsky & Cassidy, 1994; Hazan & Shaver, 1994; Jones & Cunningham, 1996). They feel threatened by separation and autonomy and deeply fear abandonment (Belsky & Cassidy, 1994; Collins & Read, 1990; Jones & Cunningham, 1996). In couple relationships, anxious/ambivalent people are demanding, dependent, clinging, and jealous (Brennan & Shaver, 1993; Hazan & Shaver, 1987, 1994; Sharpsteen & Kirkpatrick, 1997).

As indicated, individuals with insecure styles (anxious/ambivalent and avoidant) may have severe difficulties in coping with the strain involved in recovery from drug use. Examination of the impact of spousal resources on parenting patterns showed evidence concerning two of the main pairings of attachment styles among our participants: spouses with secure and avoidant attachment styles (34% of the pairs), mostly with secure wives and avoidant DU husbands, and spouses with avoidant attachment style (31% of the pairs). Spouses with secure and avoidant styles combine a secure spouse who offers support, mutuality, and intimacy with an avoidant spouse who demonstrates aloof independence, indifference to family confrontations or conflicts, who may evade parental responsibilities (Finzi, Cohen, & Ram, 2000). The avoidant DU is likely to deny the pain caused to the family by his addiction or to minimize its impact on the children, while the secure wife is probably investing her utmost in maintaining the well-being of the children and supporting the recovery process of her husband. By being aware of the children's needs, the secure wife probably tries to motivate the avoidant husband to meet his parental commitments (Finzi, Cohen, & Ram, 2000).

The relationships between spouses with avoidant attachment styles tend to be distant and aloof, allowing each partner to enjoy a sense of control over the level of proximity. Feelings of injury or rejection may trigger rage in both partners, to the point of verbal abuse or physical violence. None of them is ready to invest the effort required to rebuild the relationship. Because of lack of empathy for the children's needs, the parents may disregard their stress or suffering (Finzi, Cohen, & Ram, 2000). This type of partnership may not contain the supportive features or mutual concern required for a successful recovery process, or the ability to offer their children the special care they require.

A small number of wives who were characterized by the anxious/ambivalent attachment style (3.6%) can be described as co-dependent, to use a term that is common in referring to spousal relationships in the DU family. The non-DU spouse supplants preoccupation with her anguish by preoccupation with the addict's needs (Cullan & Carr, 1999). This preoccupation enables many to feel needed and loved, but it also enables them to avoid mature intimacy in the relationships (Favorini, 1995). Denial, splitting, projection, and identification are described as the mechanisms of the co-dependent spouse (Johnson, 1998). This type of relationship may be typical of the anxious/ambivalent partner, who tends to focus on the need for proximity, and whose sense of identity is derived from being loved and needed within the blurred boundaries of relationships (Belsky & Cassidy, 1994). This type of relationship may jeopardize the rehabilitation process (Favorini, 1995; Schlesinger & Horberg, 1990) because the sense of identity of the non-DU-spouse derives from her caretaker's role (Cullan & Carr, 1999; Haaken, 1990). The ineffectiveness of co-dependent partners, which stems from an attempt to control the adverse behavior of an afflicted (in this case, addicted) partner, may reinforce and perpetuate the undesirable behavior (Le-Poire, Hallett, & Giles, 1998).

Children's Attachment Styles

Our findings regarding the children's attachment styles were somewhat unexpected: 61.8% of them were classified as secure, 21.8% as avoidant, and 16.4% as anxious/ambivalent. Ronding et al. (1989) described a group of 18-month old prenatally drug-exposed children with secure attachment style (39% of their sample) as frail, maintaining less robust secure organization than expected. We suggest that some of the 61.8% secure children in this study may belong to a subgroup defined by Cook (1991) as "super kids"–resilient children with ostensibly excellent functioning who emerge from families with indistinct family boundaries (Bekir et al., 1993).

The correlation analyses points to links between family dimensions (cohesion and adaptability) and children's attachment styles, while the hierarchic regressions emphasize the contribution of parental attachment styles to those of the children. The relationships between the non-addicted mother and the child should also be considered. Although the mother may be in a state of psychological distress, she may provide a barrier against the negative effect of the addicted father on the psychosocial development of the child. Secure attachment style of parents has been found to predict their sensitivity, warmth, and supportiveness toward the children (Berlin & Cassidy, 1999). The majority (53.6%) of the mothers were characterized by a secure attachment style, which enabled them to provide positive parenting under varying degrees of daily parenting stress. The data concerning the association between the attachment styles of the parents and their children seem to corroborate prior theoretical and empirical studies (Berlin & Cassidy, 1999; Mikulincer & Florian, 1999). Thus, secure maternal attachment predicts secure attachment in the children, while an insecure maternal attachment (avoidant and anxious/ambivalent attachment) yields a negative correlation with the children's secure attachment. Moreover, anxious/ambivalent attachment style among DU fathers predicts the same style in their offspring. Difficulties in self-regulation typical of persons with an anxious/ambivalent style may cause DU fathers to seek their children's support, intensifying the anxiety of the children (Mikulincer, Florian, & Tolmacz, 1990). Surprisingly, paternal avoidant style correlated with secure attachment style in children, suggesting that lower involvement of DU fathers in their children's upbringing may reduce the detrimental consequences of drug use on the children (Finzi, Cohen, & Ram, 2000).

LIMITATIONS OF THE STUDY

Our research examined the impact of the fathers' drug use and of the family characteristics on the children at a specific point in time during recovery, after detoxification. Thus, these subjects do not represent the general population of DUs, and therefore the implications of living in a drug-use environment for the children's emotional state cannot be easily generalized. The small sample also limits the scope of our conclusions, and further follow-up investigation on a larger population is warranted.

Assessment of the impact of paternal drug-use on developmental outcomes in children was limited to attachment styles. Further research is needed to enhance our understanding of other personality traits such as affect regulation, defense mechanisms, and resiliency, of specific symptomatology, and of other parental characteristics.

IMPLICATIONS FOR CLINICAL PRACTICE

Following the detoxification program, DUs remain vulnerable to many daily difficulties. Such vulnerability may be exacerbated by the family environment and by patterns of interaction. Therefore, family interventions aimed at reorganizing dysfunctional relationships, roles, and boundaries are most important (Isaacson, 1991; Lavve & Altus, 2001).

Our study examined the link between personality and systemic family variables. The attachment styles of family members may portray the familial interaction and characterize the way individuals within the family manage stressful situations, interact with their spouse, and carry out parental functions.

The wife/mother is burdened with an intensive functional and emotional load. She must support her spouse, look after her children's well-being, and at the same time uphold family cohesiveness and adaptability. In the sub-spousal system, she must enable her husband to regain the bond, intimacy, warmth, and support that were neglected when he was addicted to drugs. Re-establishment of the parental sub-system within the context of a new division of roles, and a satisfactory relationship between the father and his children are also needed. Understanding the attachment styles of DUs and their wives, and understanding family dynamics can enable clinicians to evaluate the personal resources of family members and their abilities to cope with the difficult rehabilitation period. The potential for mutual support is higher in spouses characterized by a secure attachment style. In contrast, drug users and spouses characterized by insecure attachment styles are likely to have difficulties in handling the challenges arising during the recovery process and in forming the therapeutic bond necessary for further interventions promoting abstinence.

Our results indicate that a secure maternal attachment style predicts a similar attachment style among children. We suggest that maternal functioning is crucial in families with a drug-using father. A secure maternal attachment style promotes healthy development of the children and relatively adequate coping with the stressful family atmosphere. Thus it is crucial to strengthen the parenting of the non-addicted parent. Adequate maternal functioning can serve as a barrier against a tendency to role-reversal, especially among drug-user fathers characterized by an anxious/ambivalent style. A mother with a secure attachment style is equipped with more personality resources than one with an insecure attachment style; the latter is likely to have difficulties coping with the family and parental tasks required during the reorganization of the family after detoxification. Professional assistance (individual, spousal, or familial) is recommended to strengthen these women in their complex encounters. Women characterized by a secure attachment style might be able to utilize interventions using advice and support, while women with an insecure attachment styles (whose children, according to our findings, have similar attachment styles), may require a more intensive treatment in order to aid the personal and social development of their children. Interventions of this nature are likely to improve the efficacy of drug treatment programs and contribute to the well being of the drug user himself, of his family, and of the children.

CONCLUSION

In this preliminary study, the association between the attachment styles of the parents and of their children was examined. It revealed the importance of the effect of the secure maternal attachment style on the child's development. Future investigations should examine the variables of parental functioning and attitudes, their association with parental attachment styles, and their impact on the child's development. The current findings about children's attachment styles call for further examination of the risk for later developmental impairments. Longitudinal studies are needed to evaluate the children's functioning in adolescence, because this subgroup is found to be at high-risk for drug addiction and behavioral problems. Our results indicate that children exposed to parental drug use can be expected to have a better prognosis when the DU is the father and the mother has adequate parenting capacity.

REFERENCES

Ainsworth, M.D.S. (1989). Attachment beyond infancy. *American Psychologist*, 44, 709-716.

Ainsworth, M.D.S., Blehar, M.C., Waters, E., & Wall, S. (1978). *Patterns of attachment: A psychological study of the strange situation*. Hillsdale, NJ: Erlbaum.

Bartholomew K. (1997). Adult attachment processes: Individual and couple perspectives. *British Journal of Medical Psychology*, 70, 249-263.

Bekir, P., McLellan, T., Childress, R.A., & Gariti, P. (1993). Role reversals in families of substance misusers: A transgenerational phenomenon. *The International Journal of the Addictions*, 28, 613-630.

Belsky, J., & Cassidy, J. (1994). Attachment and close relationships: An individual-difference perspective. *Psychological Inquiry*, 5, 27-30.

Berlin, L.J., & Cassidy, J. (1999). Relations among relationships. In J. Cassidy & P.R. Shaver (Eds.), *Handbook of attachment: Theory, research and clinical applications*, (pp. 688-712). New York: Guilford.

Birnbaum, G.E., Orr, I., Mikulincer, M., & Florian, V. (1997). When marriage breaks up–Does attachment styles contribute to coping and mental health? *Journal of Social & Personal Relationships*, 14, 643-654.

Bowlby, J. (1973). *Attachment and loss: Separation, anxiety, and anger*. London: Hogarth Press.

Bowlby, J. (1977). The making and breaking of affectional bonds. *British Journal of Psychiatry*, 130, 201-210.

Bowlby, J. (1988). Developmental psychiatry comes to age. *American Journal of Psychiatry*, 145, 1-10.

Brennan, K.A., & Shaver, P.R. (1993). Attachment styles and parental divorce. *Journal of Divorce & Remarriage*, 21, 161-175.

Bretherton, I., Ridgeway, D., & Cassidy, J. (1990). Assessing internal working models of the attachment relationship. In M.T. Greenberg, D. Cicchetti, & E.M. Cummings (Eds.), *Attachment in the preschool years* (pp. 273-308). Chicago: The University of Chicago Press.

Byng-Hall, J. (1999). Family and couple therapy. In J. Cassidy & P.R. Shaver (Eds.), *Handbook of attachment: Theory, research, and clinical applications*, (pp. 625-645). New York: Guilford.

Clark, D.B., Moss, H.B., Kirisci, L., Mezzich, A.C., Miles, R., & Ott, P. (1997). Psychopathology in preadolescent sons of fathers with substance use disorder. *Journal of the American Academy of Child & Adolescent Psychiatry*, 36, 495-502.

Cohen, Cowan, Cowan, & Pearson (1992). Mother's and father's working models of childhood attachment relationships, parenting styles, and child behavior. *Development & Psychopathology*, 4, 417-431.

Collins, N.L., & Read, S.J. (1990). Adult attachment, working models, and relationship quality in dating couples. *Journal of Personality & Social Psychology*, 58, 644-663.

Cook, R.D. (1991). Shame, attachment, and addictions: Implications for family therapist. *Contemporary Family Therapy*, 13, 405-419.

Crnkovic, A.E., & DelCampo, R.L. (1998). A system approach to the treatment of chemical addiction. *Contemporary Family Therapy*, 20, 25-36.

Cullan, J., & Carr, A. (1999). Codependent relating: An empirical study from systemic perspective. *Contemporary Family Therapy*, 21, 505-526.

Diehl, M., Elnick, A.B., Bourbeau, I.S., & Labouvie-Vief, G. (1998). Adult attachment styles: Their relations to family context and personality. *Journal of Personality & Social Psychology*, 74, 1656-1669.

Dore, M.M. (1995). Identifying substance abuse in maltreating in families: A child welfare challenge. *Child Abuse & Neglect*, 19, 531-543.

Dore, D.D., Kauffman, E., Nelson-Zlupko, L., & Granfort, E. (1996). Psychosocial functioning and treatment needs of latency-age children from drug-involved families. *Families in Society*, 38, 595-603.

Famularo, R., Kinscherff, R., & Fenton, T. (1992). Parental substance abuse and the nature of child maltreatment. *Child Abuse & Neglect*, 16, 475-483.

Favorini, A. (1995). Concept of codependency: Blaming the victim or pathway to recovery? *Social Work*, 40, 827-830

Feeney, J.A. (1996). Attachment, caregiving, and marital satisfaction. *Personal Relationships*, 3, 401-416.

Finzi, R., Har-Even, D., Weizman, A., Tyano, S., & Shnit, D. (1996). The adaptation of the attachment style questionnaire for latency-aged children. [Hebrew]. *Psychology*, 5, 167-177.

Finzi, R., Cohen, O., & Ram, A. (2000). Attachment and divorce. *Journal of Family Psychotherapy*, 11, 1-20.

Friedman, A.S., Utada, A., & Morrissey, M.R. (1987). Families of adolescent drug abusers are "rigid": Are these families either "disengaged" or "enmeshed" or both? *Family Process*, 26, 131-148.

Gabel, S., & Shindledecker, R. (1992). Incarceration in parents of day hospital youth: Relation to parental drug substance abuse and suspected child abuse/maltreatment. *International Journal of Partial Hospitalization*, 8, 77-87.

Garbarino, J., & Vondra, J. (1987). Psychological maltreatment: Issues and perspective. In: M.R. Brassard, R. Germain, & S.N. Hart (Eds.), *Psychological maltreatment of children and youth* (pp. 24-44). New York: Pergamon Press.

George, C., & Solomon, J. (1999). Attachment and caregiving. In J. Cassidy & P.R. Shaver (Eds.), *Handbook of attachment: Theory, research, and clinical implications* (pp. 649-670). New York: Guilford.

Haaken, J. (1990). A critical analysis of the codependency construct. *Psychiatry, 53,* 396-406.

Hazan, C., & Shaver, P. (1987). Romantic love conceptualized as an attachment process. *Journal of Personality & Social Psychology,* 52, 511-524.

Hazan, C., & Shaver, P. (1994). Attachment as an organizational framework for research on close relationships. *Psychological Inquiry,* 5, 1-22.

Hofler, D.Z., & Kooyman, M. (1996). Attachment transition, addiction and therapeutic bonding–An integrative approach. *Journal of Substance Abuse Treatment,* 13, 511-519.

Hogan, D.M. (1998). Annotation: The psychological development and welfare of children of opiate and cocaine users: Review and research needs. *Journal of Child Psychology, Psychiatry, & Allied Disciplines,* 39, 609-620.

Isaacson, E.B. (1991). Chemical addiction: Individuals and family systems. *Journal of Chemical Dependency Treatment,* 4, 7-27.

Johnson, B. (1998). The mechanism of codependence in the prescription of benzodiazepines to patients with addiction. *Psychiatric Annals,* 28, 166-171.

Jones, J.T., & Cunningham, J.D. (1996). Attachment styles and other predictors of relationship satisfaction in dating couples. *Personal Relationships,* 3, 387-399.

Kang, S.Y., Kleinman, P.H., Todd, T., & Kemp, J. (1991). Familial and individual functioning in a sample of adult cocaine abusers. *Journal of Drug Issues,* 21, 579- 592.

Kobak, R.R., & Hazan, C. (1991). Attachment in marriage: Effects of security and accuracy of working models. *Journal of Personality & Social Psychology,* 60, 861- 869.

Kovacs, M. (1992). *Children's Depression Inventory.* New York and Ontario: Multi Health Systems, Inc.

Lavee, Y., & Altus, D. (2001). Family relationships as a predictor of post-treatment drug-abuse relapse: A follow-up study of drug addicts and their spouses. *Contemporary Family Therapy,* 23, 513-530.

Le-Poire, B., Hallett, J.S., & Giles, H. (1998). Codependence: The paradoxical nature of the functional-afflicted relationship. In B.H. Spitzberg, & W.R. Cupach (Eds.), *The dark side of close relationships* (pp. 153-176). Mahwah, NJ: Erlbaum.

MacKensen, G., & Cottone, R.R. (1992). Family structural issues and chemical dependency: A review of the literature from 1985 to 1991. *American Journal of Family Therapy,* 20, 227-241.

Marvin, R.S., & Stewart, R.B. (1990). A family system framework for the study of attachment. In M.T. Greenberg, D. Cicchetti, & E.M. Cummings (Eds.), *Attachment in the preschool years: Research and intervention* (pp. 51-86). Chicago: University of Chicago Press.

Meyers, S.A. (1998). Personality correlates of adult attachment style. *Journal of Social Psychology,* 133, 407-409.

Milkulincer, M., & Florian, V. (1999). The association between spouses' self reports of attachment styles and representations of family dynamic. *Family Process,* 38, 69-83.

Milkulincer, M., Florian, V., & Tolmacz, R. (1990). Attachment styles and fear of personal death: A case study of affect regulation. *Journal of Personality & Social Psychology,* 58, 273-280.

Mikulincer, M., & Nachson, O. (1991). Attachment styles and patterns of self-disclosure. *Journal of Personality & Social Psychology,* 61, 321-331.

Mikulincer, M. (1995). Attachment style and the mental representation of the self. *Journal of Personality & Social Psychology*, 69, 1203-1215.

Mikulincer, M. (1997). Adult attachment style and information processing: Individual differences in curiosity and cognitive closure. *Journal of Personality & Social Psychology*, 72, 1217-1230.

National Center on Child Abuse and Neglect (NCCAN) (1994). *Protecting children in substance-abusing families*. Washington, DC: Department of Health and Human Services.

Olson, D.H. (1986). Circumplex model: VII: Validation studies and FACES III. *Family Process*, 25, 337-351.

Pfeffer, C., Lipkins, R., Plutchik, R., & Mizruchi, M.S. (1988). Normal children at risk for suicide: Two-year follow-up study. *Journal of the American Academy of Child & Adolescent Psychiatry*, 27, 34-41.

Pistole, C.M. (1989). Attachment in adult romantic relationships: Style of conflict resolution and relationship satisfaction. *Journal of Social Personal Relationships*, 6, 505-510.

Plasse, B.R. (1995). Parenting groups for recovering addicts in a day treatment center. *Social Work*, 40, 65-74.

Rivinus, T.,M., Levoy, D., Matzko, M., & Seifer, R. (1992). Hospitalized children of substance abusing parents and physically and sexually abused children: A comparison. *Journal of the American Academy of Child & Adolescent Psychiatry*, 31, 1019-1023.

Ronding, C., Beckwith, L., & Howard, J. (1989). Characteristics of attachment organization and play organization in prenatally drug-exposed toddlers. *Development and Psychopathology*, 1, 277-289.

Rusbult, C.E., Verette, J., Whitney, G.A., Solvik, L.F., & Lipkus, I. (1991). Accommodation process in close relationships: Theory and preliminary empirical evidence. *Journal of Personality & Social Psychology*, 60, 53-78.

Scherling, D. (1994). Prenatal cocaine exposure and childhood psychopathology: A developmental analysis. *American Journal of Orthopsychiatry*, 64, 9-21.

Schlesinger, S.E., & Horberg, L.K. (1990). Comprehensive treatment of addictive families. *Psychology of Addictive Behaviors*, 4, 26-30.

Senchak, M., & Leonard, K.E. (1992). Attachment styles and marital adjustment among newlywed couples. *Journal of Social & Personal Relationships,* 9, 51-64.

Sharpsteen, D.J., & Kirkpatrick, L.A. (1997). Romantic jealousy and adult romantic attachment. *Journal of Personality & Social Psychology*, 72, 627-640.

Sheridan, M.J. (1995). A proposal intergenerational model of substance abuse, family functioning, and abuse/neglect. *Child Abuse & Neglect*, 19, 519-530.

Simpson, J.A., & Rholes, W.S. (1998). Attachment in adulthood. In J.A. Simpson & W.S. Rholes (Eds.), *Attachment theory and close relationships* (pp. 3-21). New York: Guilford Press.

Spielberger, C.D., Edwards, C.D., Lushene, R.E., Montuori, J., & Platzek, D. (1973). *Preliminary test manual for the State-Trait Anxiety Inventory for Children*. Palo Alto, CA: Consulting Psychologists Press.

Teichman, M., & Basha, U. (1996). Codependency and family cohesion and adaptability: Changes during treatment in therapeutic community. *Substance Use and Misuse*, 31, 599-615.

Teichman, U., & Navon, S. (1990). Family evaluation: The circumplex model [in Hebrew]. *Psychologia, 2,* 36-46.

Wilens, T.E., Biederman, J., Kiely, K., Bredin, E., & Spencer, T.J. (1995). Pilot study of behavioral and emotional disturbances in the high-risk children of parents with opioid dependence. *Journal of the American Academy of Child and Adolescent Psychiatry, 34,* 779-785.

Weinfield, N.S., Sroufe, A.L., Egeland, B., & Carlson, E.A. (1999). The nature of individual differences in infant-caregiver attachment. In J. Cassidy & P.R. Shaver (Eds.), *Handbook of attachment: Theory, research, and clinical implications* (pp. 68-88). New York: Guilford.

Wolock, I., & Magura, S. (1996). Parental substance abuse as predictor of child maltreatment. Re-report. *Child Abuse & Neglect, 20,* 1183-1193.

Social Support:
A Key to Positive Parenting Outcomes
for Mothers in Residential Drug Treatment
with Their Children

Josephine Y. Wong

SUMMARY. This study explored parenting experiences of ten mothers residing with their young children in four residential drug treatment facilities in New York City and how these experiences related to the perceived support of the social environment of the facility. Through the lenses of the self-in-relations theory and family-centered service model, the study examined the supportive function of the treatment program including the program structure, the staff, and fellow mothers in affecting the mothers' parenting experience and outcomes. Programmatic, policy, and research implications of the study's findings are discussed. *[Article copies available for a fee from The Haworth Document Delivery Service: 1-800-HAWORTH. E-mail address: <docdelivery@ haworthpress.com> Website: <http://www.HaworthPress.com> © 2006 by The Haworth Press, Inc. All rights reserved.]*

Josephine Y. Wong, PhD, MSW, R-CSW, is Policy and Planning Analyst, New York City Department of Mental Health (E-mail: Wong.josephine@worldent.att.net).
This paper is based on her doctoral dissertation at New York University School of Social Work.

[Haworth co-indexing entry note]: "Social Support: A Key to Positive Parenting Outcomes for Mothers in Residential Drug Treatment with Their Children." Wong, Josephine Y. Co-published simultaneously in *Journal of Social Work Practice in the Addictions* (The Haworth Press, Inc.) Vol. 6, No. 1/2, 2006, pp. 113-137; and: *Impact of Substance Abuse on Children and Families: Research and Practice Implications* (ed: Shulamith Lala Ashenberg Straussner, and Christine Huff Fewell) The Haworth Press, Inc., 2006, pp. 113-137. Single or multiple copies of this article are available for a fee from The Haworth Document Delivery Service [1-800-HAWORTH, 9:00 a.m. - 5:00 p.m. (EST). E-mail address: docdelivery@haworthpress.com].

Available online at http://www.haworthpress.com/web/JSWPA
doi:10.1300/J160v06n01_06

KEYWORDS: Parenting, residential drug treatment, social support, women, relational theories

INTRODUCTION

Women who are in residential drug treatment with their children reside in a highly-structured social environment. Assuming an active parenting role while participating in treatment can be demanding. The challenge can be exacerbated by the women's frequent insufficient and/or inadequate parenting skills (Daghastani, 1988; Greenleaf, 1989), negative perceptions of their parenting role by others (Finkelstein, 1994; Smyth & Miller, 1997), and their shame-filled, guilt-ridden, negative parental self (Finkelstein, 1994; Sterk-Eifson, 1998; Van-Bremen & Chasnoff, 1994). The negative parental self in conjunction with the negative parenting experience impacts the substance-abusing mothers' perception of themselves and their relationship with their children and others. Parental self-concept, necessary for effective parenting, consists of a combination of experiences from one's own childhood, as well as current experiences with parenting (Benedek, 1956, 1959, 1970; Davis, 1990; Demick, Bursik & Diabiase, 1993). In the case of women in residential drug treatment with their children, their current parenting experiences take place within the social environment of a mother-child drug treatment facility.

Social support can facilitate the expression of parenting behavior (i.e., an improved adjustment to the parenting role, an increased ability to express empathy, and a secure feeling of being a parent) that is conducive to a child's healthy development (Ainsworth, 1968; Winnicott, 1987). However, social support can only be effective when perceived as helpful (Gottlieb, 1981, 1983; Oakley, 1992), and a social environment can be a source of stress as well as support (Belsky, 1984; Belsky & Vondra, 1989). Substance-abusing mothers' multi-faceted problems in their lives (e.g., receiving inadequate parenting as a child, being a victim of abuses, having received little social support from spouses or partners, having unmet dependency needs, feelings of powerlessness, depression and other mental disorders) shape their experience with and their expectation of support (Mayes, 1995, Well & Jackson, 1992). Indeed, substance-abusing mothers can be hesitant in seeking social support, even when they are already in contact with helping professionals (Taylor, 1993; VanBremen & Chasnoff, 1994). Hence, the family-centered model advocates for enhancing the supportive function of a family's social environment by service providers (Dunst & Trivette, 1988; Dunst, Trivette, & Thompson, 1990). However, the social support function of the social environment of a residential treatment program for mothers and children has never been examined comprehensively. This study explored how mothers who were in residential drug treatment with their children experienced parenting and how those experiences related to their perceived social support provided by the program structure, the staff, and fellow mothers.

REVIEW OF LITERATURE

During the past decade, treatment models have gradually become more responsive to substance-abusing women's parenting needs along with their treatment needs (Luthar & Walsh, 1995; Uziel-Miller et al., 1998; VanBremen & Chasnoff, 1994; Yaffe, Jenson, & Howard, 1995; Zelvin, 1997). Children are allowed to stay with their mothers by some residential drug treatment programs to remove treatment barriers–fear of loss of child custody and lack of a support network to provide childcare (Goldberg, 1995; Goldberg et al., 1996; Well & Jackson, 1992). Although the majority of the residential drug treatment programs for women employ a Therapeutic Community model (Times, Jainchill, & Deleon, 1994), self-in-relation theories have been adopted experimentally in the design of some programs for women and their children (Byington, 1993, 1997; Finkelstein, 1993; Luther & Walsh, 1995). This model is based on the belief that addictions represent, at least in part, a misplaced striving for connection, and that it is the disconnection from others that leads to a sense of isolation in women and to their substance abuse. Consequently, substance-abusing mothers working toward recovery must learn to build and rebuild a healthy relationship with themselves and with other people–one that is reciprocal and that facilitates the development of self-esteem and a positive sense of self. In this light, in addition to needing child-care and parenting skills to maintain basic parenting function while in treatment, these mothers require social support to build their relational self, including their parental self.

There is limited literature on the relationship between the social support provided by the social environment of the treatment facility, the manner in which this support is provided, perceived, and received by the mothers, and the parenting experience of the mothers in residence. Moreover, the few treatment options and inflexibility in the treatment approach have resulted in narrow treatment outcome measures (Goldberg, 1995; LaFave & Desporates Echols, 1999). Parenting outcome measures have been limited to the parenting component of treatment programs (Camp & Finkelstein, 1997; Uziel-Miller, 1998). Programmatic constraints such as lack of funding, little staff training, and liability issues applicable to providing services to children may also contributed to insufficient attention to the mothers' parenting experiences while in the treatment. Moreover, studies of residential drug treatment program for women and their children measure outcomes in a structured way, without providing much contextual, process-oriented understanding of the social dynamics that take place in the treatment setting and their possible impact on treatment outcomes (Brown, Melchoir, Waite-Obrien, & Huba, 2002; Conners, Bradley, Whiteside-Mansell, & Crone, 2001). Such studies provide limited insight into what specifically can be done to enhance the social support functions of these programs.

METHOD

This study used an exploratory-descriptive design since not much is known about substance abusing mothers, their perception of social support from the social environment of the treatment program (the program structure, staff and fellow mothers), and related parenting experience. This study employed a combined qualitative and quantitative method–the QUAL-quant mode (Creswell, 1994), with the qualitative method being the dominant study design. Strengths of the combined methodology include: (1) providing two or more sources to achieve a comprehensive picture of a subject, known as "triangulation"; (2) counteracting threats to validity inherent in one method by balancing strengths and weaknesses of all measures and source of data; and (3) enhancing the likelihood of achieving completeness in portraying the context of the topic under study (Davis, 1994; Padgett, 1998).

The qualitative method, conducted through three separate interviews with each subject, sought to discover and convey the complex worlds of participants in a holistic manner using "thick description" (Padgett, 1998), and to gain an in-depth understanding of the group under study through participatory observation and intensive interviewing (Ely, Anzul, Friedman, Garner, & Steimertz, 1991). Quantitative data was collected through a Family Support Scale–a 5-point Likert Scale (Dunst, Jenkins, & Trivette, 1984) that measured the mothers' perceived social support of their social environments, plus a brief questionnaire focusing on demographics of both the mothers and children. IRB approval for this study was obtained through New York University.

PARTICIPANTS

The population under study was adult female parents who were in a New York City-based residential drug treatment program with their children. Five residential mother-child programs were identified from the New York State Office of Alcoholism and Substance Abuse Services Directory for Women's Treatment Services (1999), its on-line Provider Directory (2001), and subsequent telephone inquiries. Four programs, with capacities ranging from 12 to approximately 50 mother-child units, expressed interest in allowing the author access to their residents, who were then invited to participate in this paid study. One program allowed the mothers to be in treatment with up to three children, another program allowed two children, and two programs had a one-child admission policy. The age cut-off for the admitted child was five, with occasional exception for older children. Built upon the Therapeutic Community model, all programs offered both substance abuse treatment and parenting programming, although the programs varied from each other.

Ten mothers were recruited through nonprobability, purposive sampling (Reid & Smith, 1989). Six mothers were from the two larger programs and four from the two smaller ones. All the participants, chosen based on their capability to articulate their experience, had been in treatment for at least three months, and were between 25 and 45 years of age. Seven mothers reported to be single, two divorced or separated and one married. Eight of the ten mothers had prior drug treatment(s). Two mothers were in treatment with two children and eight with one child, although one of the eight was in the process of admitting her other child to the program. The children's ages ranged from infancy to five. Six mothers had other children in the community who were cared for by family members or in foster care. All had resumed regular contact with their children since they entered treatment.

PROCEDURE

Data was collected during Fall, 2001. A three-interview structure with three contacts over the course of 1 to 3 weeks was used. Open-ended questions within categories were asked in order to facilitate participants in reconstructing their experience (Seidman, 1998), as well as to ensure that the key domains of the study were covered (Padgett, 1998). The Family Support Scale (Dunst, Jenkins, & Trivette, 1984) and a brief demographic questionnaire were administered during the first interview. In addition, fieldnotes were created, documenting the researcher's observation, with guidelines, of what took place in the natural environment of the participants, as well as her reaction and reflection. The fieldnotes served as: (1) A triangulation tool that established mutuality between field observation and an in-depth interview to enhance the rigor of a study (Ely et al., 1991); (2) an additional source of data supplementing the contextual data from the interview (Calson et al., 1998); and (3) a self-reflective and reflexive measure to help the researcher be mindful of his/her biases (Ely et al., 1991; Padgett, 1998). The data from the ten participants provided enough information to the level of information saturation (Lincoln & Guba, 1985), repetition and redundancy of themes (Padget, 1998), and the number of participants was sufficient to reflect the range and sites that make up the population (Seidman, 1998).

Data analysis included: (1) Transcribed audiotapes of the interviews; (2) use of Open Coding–bracketing data from the transcripts that appeared meaningful; (3) identification of themes through an inductive-reductive-inductive approach (Strauss & Corbin, 1990) until reaching the point of repetitiveness and redundancy; (4) compilation of the ratings from the Family Support Scale; and (5) comparison of qualitative and quantitative findings. Furthermore, trustworthiness and vigor of the findings from qualitative data analysis were enhanced by: (1) Prolonged engagement; (2) a negative case analysis; (3) triangulation between field observation and interviews; (4) peer debriefing and support; (5) member checking; and (6) an audit trail (Padgett, 1998).

RESULTS

Both qualitative and quantitative findings were consistent in describing the treatment facilities as supportive environments.

Findings from Quantitative Data Analysis

All items on the 5-point Family Support Scale that pertain to the formal support offered by the residential drug treatment program (e.g., parent group, daycare, staff at the facility, and other mothers at the facility) were perceived as either "very helpful" (4), or "extremely helpful" (5); these perceptions were consistent regardless of the lengths of stay in the program. On the other hand, informal support networks (e.g., own parents, extended family and kin, friends or co-workers, neighbors who are parents, or church) were rated as "not available" (1), "not helpful at all" (2), or "sometimes helpful" (3). Ratings of their spouse or partner were polarized, with "not available" (1), or "not helpful at all" (2), at one end, or "extremely helpful" (5), at the other. The last response was provided by mothers with non drug-abusing spouse or partner.

Findings from Qualitative Data Analysis

There were five main themes and 23 subthemes that were identified as permeating the mothers' parenting experiences while in treatment. They can be seen in Table 1.

Theme 1: A Parenting Experience Shaped by a Parenting Desire

All ten mothers expressed a desire to parent their children, which was a determining factor in their decision to enter treatment, and in their choice and expectation of treatment.

Characterizing the decision to enter treatment. All mothers described an active decision-making process connected to two motivating factors—an effort to avoid separation from their children, regardless of the availability of childcare arrangements in the community, and a need for an external structure to facilitate their parenting. The following excerpts articulate this internal process experienced by the mothers:

> *I didn't want to bring him into this negative environment but I couldn't afford to separate from him for 15 months. When I was in a 30-day treatment, I kept five pictures of him by my bed . . . I cried a lot, a lot of guilt, so I knew how much it hurt. . . .The biggest concern was to be separated from him and traumatizing him in terms of separation. As a child, I was separated from my mother for about two years . . . and I haven't gotten over it . . . and I didn't want him to call my mother Mommy.*

> *I was fighting for (my son) . . . They didn't give me visitation until I had proof that I was coming into this program . . . I knew I could*

not do it outpatient because I would be out there and need the drug. Now I want him in my life; I just don't know how I can do drugs and be a good parent.

Shaping their expectations for support in treatment. The children's stay in the treatment facility affected the mothers' treatment expectation; most of the mothers voiced a need for a more family-focused approach: "I was imagining a little house for mothers and kids . . . I volunteered to come, so I had expected a more gentle environment." "There is not a lot of child's program and they need to consider that . . . To overlook what's written and look at us individually." "I'm talking about the things that she's growing up and doing now. She's exploring her body. We don't have parenting classes like that."

TABLE 1. Themes and Subthemes of Mother's Parenting Experiences while in Treatment

THEMES	SUBTHEMES
A parenting experience shaped by a parenting desire	• Characterizing the decision to enter treatment • Shaping their expectations for support in treatment
Coping with ambivalence concerning support received in treatment	• Overcoming shame and powerlessness • Trust at one's own pace • Searching for safety • Seeking validation of the self
Developing a new parenting experience: Stepping out of the shadow of guilt	• Confronting the guilt • Counteracting the guilt
Significance of support: Sustaining and containing the mother through treatment	• Serving as a protective shield • Building a foundation in their lives • Providing safety for self-exploration • Offering empathic attunement • Meeting parenting needs • Enhancing self-development • Facilitating an integration of the good and bad parental self • Fostering an integration of the different aspects of the self • Cultivating mother-to-mother support
Transformed relationships: Nature, perception, and approach	• An emerging maternal empathy • Openness and honesty in communication • Taking risk to trust • Improved self-esteem • A clearer boundary between self and others • Taking part in constructive relationship-building

Theme 2: Coping with Ambivalence Concerning Support Received in Treatment

Having been denied the opportunity as a child to learn appropriate support-seeking behavior or to connect to responsive people, the mothers developed minimal expectation about social support, as well as ambivalence about seeking it. However, the findings revealed that the ambivalence could be addressed and overcome in a supportive or a holding environment (Winicott, 1965, 1971, 1987).

Overcoming shame and powerlessness. All ten mothers viewed being attended to and listened to as supportive. The mothers placed a higher value on how the staff related to them, rather than on what the staff said or did. They appreciated the staff's openness, caring, accessibility, identification with them, and respect for their individualities. In response, the mothers gradually shared their stories, thoughts, and feelings. One mother narrated:

> *(My mother) sent me outside when she smoked marijuana, no matter what the weather condition was . . . she didn't like me to cry and she would hit me . . . I kept my feelings inside, believing that it didn't matter, I didn't matter . . . Here, (the staff) did not make up things or lie to me. They are open with you. We can tell them how they made us feel. They will apologize to you and say, "I'm wrong," even in front of others at House Meetings.*

However, feeling ashamed, guilty, and inadequate as a parent, the mothers needed to confront their ambivalence in seeking support. One mother recalled:

> *I went to feed my son everyday when he was in the hospital but I felt strange. . . . I was escorted in there . . . I knew I messed up, I was using drugs . . . I couldn't take my baby with me. I was just feeling strange when I was feeding him . . . when everybody knew that I had messed up, like "here's the mother who's on drugs.". . . (After 20 months in this program), in public (before the staff and other mothers), I have to put my foot down when my son doesn't listen because it is really embarrassing.*

Trust at one's own pace. The mothers attempted to develop trust in the staff, at their own comfort level and pace, although they came from backgrounds where they were taught not to trust. The data suggested that the mothers' hunger for a trusting object and their positive experience with certain helpful and caring professionals through the otherwise overwhelming program admission process and a difficult treatment process had, in part, accounted for the development of trust. Some mothers were trusting enough to rely on the staff to regulate their emotions and to develop a positive sense of self, as exemplified in the following excerpt:

> *The psychologist is great . . . When I was crying so much and feeling so down, she said that was a "break through." I said it was a little nervous "break down". . . but I snapped out of it. . . . If I would talk about things, I would rather talk to a staff, somebody who can help me through, because I'm very emotional. I trust them.*

Searching for safety. How the facility responded to the mothers' safety concerns affected the mothers' trust of the program. In addition, some of the mothers' safety concerns appeared to be connected to their past experience of parenting or being parented.

> *Given where we were coming from, being an addict and all that . . . some of us even have mental difficulties, this is probably the best place to learn not to react physically toward our children. . . . Five days a week you can talk to somebody who knows a lot about kids . . .*

Seeking Validation of the Self. Validation of their emotions and experience, as well as of the intrinsic values of their selves, the parental self in particular, was reported by both the staff and other mothers. "My mother used to call me a liar! I never talked about the abuse or my daughter's death until I came (to this program), then I let the tears go." "My mother did not like me to cry and she would hit me, I learned that I didn't matter . . . I just felt dirty, disgusted, nasty about the rape . . . (my counselor) accepted who I am and I started to have my own values (of myself)."

The parenting by fellow mothers at times triggered memories and associated negative feelings in some mothers as to how they, as children, were treated by their own mothers. Nevertheless, the mothers found each other supportive. "It is basically up to us to give ourselves the help that we need. The staff is here to supervise all that." "After all these years of isolation, we cried and laughed together." The positive responses they offered each other were emotionally empowering, resulting in their ability and willingness to "give back."

Theme 3: Developing a New Parenting Experience–Stepping Out of the Shadow of Guilt

When describing their parenting experiences in the treatment, all ten mothers consistently reported mixed emotions. While a gratifying experience and positive parental self were being formulated, the mothers' guilt and anxiety were also activated. Yet, there was an emerging integration between the two aspects of the parental self over time.

Confronting the Guilt. All mothers reported experiencing a heightened sense of guilt related to their parenting. This resulted partly from reflecting on their prior struggles with fulfilling parenting responsibilities and living a "drugging" life, and partly from the uneasiness of assuming parenting responsibilities in the environment of a residential drug treatment program. Two mothers revealed this internal process:

> *I am now aware of how bad my daughter's asthma is. But when I was getting high, the signs, symptoms, I didn't notice it, I didn't try to notice it.*

> *I'm happy that (my son) is so little . . . basically he has no idea what's going on around him, he's not gonna hold resentment against me when he's big; he's not going to remember (having been in this place).*

In addition, the mothers felt that their parenting was under close scrutiny and supervision, which made many of them feel like "a child with a child." This feeling, when not handled with sensitivity by the program and its staff, activated their sense of inadequacy, and intensified their guilt and shame. "I would like to say parenting is easier because you can get help 7 days a week. But it's not because you're under someone else's watch."

Simultaneously, a bonding experience with their children in the treatment facility had enabled them to perceive their children in a more positive light or within the child's developmental and social context, leading to greater feelings of guilt. One mother reflected:

> *My older daughter is mad at me sometimes . . . I am a different parent (now), I attend to them more and say "no" to them more . . .*

also, there are a lot of things in here that I can't do with her. But she doesn't understand.

Counteracting the Guilt. All ten mothers reported joy and success in their current parenting, which mitigated their parental guilt. The mothers experienced significant emotional support by the simple presence of their children, valued the chance–some considered it their "second chance" or "last chance"–to be a parent. The child's presence provided the mother with a base to build on her parenting experience, develop her parenting skills and her parental self. All mothers acknowledged improved parenting skills, and expressed an urgency and high motivation to learn and experiment with ways to interact effectively with their children as they were growing and developing in the mothers' presence. These positive experiences aided in countering their negative parental self. "I am doing normal parenting, not bad parenting." "I'm a better mother than my mother was to me. What she didn't do for her kids, I have to do more for my kids."

Theme 4: The Power of Support–Sustaining and Containing the Mothers Through Treatment

Support provided by the treatment facility reportedly buffered the multiple stresses that the mothers were experiencing in residential treatment with their children. The described stresses included: maintaining sobriety; communal living; adjusting to the program structure; coping with parental guilt and anxiety; and meeting the program's high demands for participation in both treatment and parenting programmings: "I'm surprised that I can make it this far, it's an experience colored with guilt"; "My child and I tough it out together"; "I had preconceived prejudice about being here but it turned out to be a great experience."

Serving as a protective shield. The residency in the therapeutic community created a protective shield for the mothers from their original communities, in which they had juggled with fulfilling parenting responsibilities, living a "drugging life," and engaged in many abusive and unhealthy relationships. The mothers felt the therapeutic community offered them the opportunity to be a parent and to focus on their parenting. As one mother put it, "Here I can give my children the undivided attention that they need, not like a robot; pick them up, do (the task) and put them down. Don't hear them, don't talk to them." In addition, the setting awarded them a safe place to experience healthy relationships and to heal from social sanctions to which these mothers had been subjected in the course of developing their parental self.

Building a foundation in their lives. The program structure was viewed by some mothers as building a foundation in their lives, which they had lacked. More important, many mothers understood that being protected did not mean being freed from the responsibilities or natural consequences of their behavior inherent in the Therapeutic Community Model. On the contrary, as they progressed, they showed increased receptiveness to the external structure. As a mother put it,

> *This environment is protective. It's not like I was living with my mother. Here, I can't get away with things. . . . In here, I can't run from treatment while I am in treatment.*

The self-identified choice of and readiness for treatment, and a desire to be with the child had made the mothers more willing partners, which then minimized their previous psychological barriers of responding to treatment. "I was doing it for others; I had to wait till I know it's time for me to do it." "I didn't get anything out of (the previous treatment) because I wasn't receptive to it, I was not open. But now I wanted to come."

Providing safety for self exploration. Several mothers perceived the program structure and the residency as providing their family with a sense of routine, predictability, and safety that had been missing in their lives. "I can see them everyday. I know I will pick them up at 3:00 in the daycare and they know I will be there," a mother expressed. Partaking in planning their weekend activities in the community made them feel safe. In addition, this new behavior had been incorporated into some mothers' own coping outside. "I'll call my mother if I would be five minutes late because I was expected to do so in this program."

Feeling safe, the mothers began to self-examine, reach out to learn, and to relate. They felt they could explore and afford to make mistakes, a reflection of an initial development of the true self–a self that feels alive and real (Winnicott, 1960, 1971). "Because this place is a safe haven, I can start confronting issues that I've never done in my entire life, with the support of the staff, before I go back out there to the real world." "I can go to (the staff) for help as opposed to driving myself crazy." In particular, they began to show high motivation and enthusiasm in exploring different parenting skills, overcome certain psychological barriers to their parenting role, and began to develop a positive parental self.

Offering empathic attunement. The staff members' traits or the way they related to the mothers–their ability to be attuned or empathic to the mothers, or their simple, non-intrusive presence–were considered supportive. "Not that they solved anything, but they are always there. They have a lot of time and patience for me." Furthermore, the mothers saw the staff "calming" them "down"–being ego supportive–while assisting them in approaching painful issues or revisiting difficult experiences as a significant support. "My counselor knows my fears." "It's a subject that you can't go deep unless you are with your therapist."

Internalization of an empathic staff member had been a somewhat different process for different mothers, especially during the testing time of a staff's departure from his/her job, which unfortunately happened quite often. Their different responses were exemplified as follows:

> *I was very close with my counselor; I have never been this close with anybody in my life . . . (My counselor's) leaving opened me up. I'm not saying that I didn't have to work through my feelings. I went to the program director and told her how angry I was about her leaving. But after I processed it, I felt that I could deal with it. The director is a good listener; she let me talk.*

> *The staff members that I was comfortable with, they all left . . . It's sad! We don't even say goodbye sometime, we just watch the person leave.*

Meeting parenting needs. Most of the mothers gradually experienced the support of the parenting programming, which ranged from parenting class, daycare, therapeutic work, to reconnecting them with family and children living in the community. However, the mothers expressed frustration about the un-integrated parenting and drug treatment programs: they felt that insufficient time was given to be with their children, that they and their children were serviced separately for the majority of the day, that the parenting program was secondary to treatment program and less stably structured, and that they were not given sufficient power in influencing the parenting programming. Two mothers verbalized such frustration:

> *This is a parent-child program. They should consider more children programming . . . they should give more time to the parent and child, they should encourage that.*

They expect you to be so involved with parenting but didn't give you enough time . . . the children are confused as to who should they listen to–their mother or the staff?

Enhancing self-development. The mothers grew from being passive recipients into more active participants, showing an emerging ability to separate their own needs from those of others, seeking to have those needs met, and actively exploring parenting skills. In this evolving process, the mothers started to work on the unresolved negative feelings they had regarding their significant others and were also learning to form partnerships with others for the pursuit of mutual goals. Two mothers spoke of this shift:

I still love (the children's father) but right now my children come first.

Because of my anger, I've never heard my mother in this way. . . . I'm looking forward to letting my anger (at my mother) go.

Facilitating an integration of the good and bad parental self. Empathy expressed by staff members towards and validation of the mothers, either for their parenting or other aspects of their lives, was facilitative of the integration of the good and bad parental self:

I was never a daughter so it was hard to know whether I have done (the parenting) right; I have no reference . . . I thought I didn't have it in me (to be a parent) . . . I was feeling very bad with my son, thinking that God had not thought this out properly: How could he do this to this child–giving me as his mother . . . We feel bad being a parent here and their support is significant to help us through . . . I'm pretty good with parenting now and many people here are telling me (that) . . . I shared my inner struggles with the parenting teacher who assured me that I've done an excellent job as a parent, that there's no perfect parent.

Fostering an integration of the different aspects of the self. Another result of being nurtured in a holding environment was a level of integration of the different parts of the mother's self. The different roles she played–an addict, a mother, a woman, a daughter, and a worker–were no longer maintained in isolation. Rather, they began to connect.

I have to learn how to be honest to myself, especially in recovery; if I didn't admit that I did have a drug problem then I wouldn't be a mother to my son . . . I am a mother before I am, what you call it, a career woman. My child comes first, if (boyfriend) can't wait, that's his problem.

Cultivating mother-to-mother support. The isolation experienced by the mothers was broken by their mutual validation and mutual help. While some individual mothers were not seen as supportive, the entire group of mothers *was* perceived as a source of support. The women were developing the capability to identify other mothers whom they considered helpful and positive, and separating them from the entire group and from the negative aspects of the communal, T.C. living, signifying a development of the mother's own sense of self and her relationships. "Some mothers here are about games, I don't go to them." "If you persist in your old behavior and are looking for troubles, the door is closed."

It is important to note that the children's presence created new dynamics in the mothers' interactions with one another, a finding that has not been addressed in previous studies. The mothers reported that their children's presence facilitated the support of other mothers, and yet could become a source of conflict when they became entangled in their children's fights with each other.

Theme 5: Transformed Relationships–The Nature, Perception, and Approach

Through open communication and empathic interaction between the mother and those involved in the program, and through behavior consequences to negative interaction, the mothers were experiencing positive relationships, which in turn changed their perception of, behavior toward, and the nature of these relationships.

An Emerging Maternal Empathy. The mothers showed an emerging, or stronger, ability to express their empathy toward their children. They found themselves identifying with their children's needs and their emotions more easily, as they were bonding and developing a closer relationship with their children. One mother reflected: "I just wasn't very motherly; the way I just changed (her older daughter), fed her, I thought that was it. I didn't feel with her the bond that I have with my son (who is with her now), that I'll do anything I can for him."

With a stronger maternal empathy, the mothers began to perceive their children differently–more positively–which, in turn, improved the parent-child relationship, the parental self, and the parenting experience.

Openness and Honesty in Communication. Being a participant in a therapeutic community, where the community served a therapeutic function, made the mothers feel that they had received guidance in being honest with themselves and others. One mother gave the following account:

> *The first time I wrote (the proposal to move to the next level of treatment), I felt good about it. 'Cause it was like giving somebody a chance to know me better. . . . now I have to write another proposal, I have to take a look at myself again. . . . I have to dig deep, assessing how much I have grown. . . . you have to be honest because (the staff) can tell if you are not.*

Moreover, in their positive experiences with certain staff members, who had shared "a part of themselves," the mothers gradually modeled their attitudes and behaviors after the staff. A mother credited the staff: "They showed me an understanding that I needed to reach myself."

Individual therapeutic work and family counseling also played a role in fostering open and honest communication with children and family outside of the facility. "We played this game (in play therapy) about why her father is not here with her."

Taking Risk to Trust. Overall, the mothers described their relationships with staff, professional and para-professional, some of them "former" addicts, as trusting. They felt contained empathically by the professional staff and formed a mutual identification with those staff members who had a history of substance abuse because "they are not far removed . . . so they are pretty compassionate."

However, practicing honest communication with staff members in uneven power positions was a challenge when a mother and a staff member did not agree about parenting issues. While not all mothers were comfortable yet in voicing differing opinions, trust in the process and outcome of open communication was something the mothers tried to achieve. "I wasn't able to do that yet, but admired a peer who could. It takes a lot of guts to stand up to someone on staff," expressed by one mother.

Staff members who left the program created a crisis of trust and yet an opportunity for furthering that trust. Staff's willingness to address the matter could maintain the mothers' trust, and allow for the staff member to be internalized as a "good object." However, when they were feeling that the agency was handling the staff member's departure in an "underhanded," secretive manner, the mothers were unable to grow from that experience and, instead, became more distrustful.

Improved Self-Esteem. Over time, many mothers reported feeling positive about themselves as a person and a mother, moving away from the previous low self-esteem and shameful feelings. "People can trust me with a dollar or something and know that I'll come back." "I am feeling good, stronger, and I think I can help my older daughters more (who have been so supportive of me)."

A Clearer Boundary Between Self and Others. The mothers evidenced a healthier sense of self and relationships, with a clearer role/self boundary resulting in better relationships. As a mother put it:

> *In my residency here, I've learned that everything that happened in my life wasn't all my fault . . . It's about me today. I should not have to spare anybody's feelings anymore. 'Cause I think I've spared enough of mine to not to hurt them.*

This clearer boundary was noticeably reflected in the mothers' relapse prevention. While entering treatment was primarily for their children, approaching program completion, the mothers verbalized a need to work on relapse prevention for themselves not for their children or significant others. A mother pondered, "I'm not sure whether my love for my son is enough to keep me clean. I need to know how to stop for me."

Furthermore, the mothers' handling of the mixed emotions they experienced as they approached treatment completion was another indication of their maturing selves and a continuing effort to define and maintain a clearer boundary between self and others. One mother, for example, saw herself as being "in mental and emotional transition," and therefore, shifted her focus away from the program onto the community-based support.

DISCUSSION

This study's rich, contextual findings show that social support provided by different aspects of the parent-child residential drug treatment program was significant in bringing the mothers into treatment and maintaining them there despite the multi-stressors generated from assuming an active parenting role in the highly structured, congregate social environment where demand was high for participation in both treatment and parenting programming. This process resulted in a complex but rich parenting experience and an improved relationship with self, their children, and others. Alongside, a level of personal growth and self-development furthered the mothers' responsiveness to treatment.

An examination of relationship outcomes indicated that the children's presence in the program was experienced as a major support, and played a critical role in coming to the program, and in shaping their expectations for social support from the program and utilization of the support. While the desire to parent motivated the mothers into and sustained them through treatment, the empathic responses they received from the staff contained them and facilitated the development of a positive perception of themselves and their children, a mutually-enhancing relationship with their children, and a positive and more integrated parental self. Consistent with the family-centered service model (Dunst, Trivette, & Thompson, 1990; Dunst & Trivette, 1988) the experience of support from the interaction with staff members of all levels, fellow mothers and their children, as well as from the program structure and programming, provided mothers with a sense of safety and energy to reach out, explore, and grow, and became capable of providing support, including empathic response, to their children. Furthermore, the mothers took on a more mature approach in relationship building in general, which facilitated and enhanced their ability to use the social supports available to them.

As documented in the literature (Benedek, 1956, 1959; Demick, Bursik, & Diabiase, 1993), motherhood and parenthood, and the connected parental self, are a developmental stage in an adult's life. Its development is subject to the impact of the current experience and the subjective meaning and perception the mother gives to the experience. These findings suggest that mother-child treatment facilities provid not only a place for the mothers to receive substance abuse treatment and to perform parenting simultaneously (Goldberg, 1995; Goldberg et al., 1996), but also a holding, facilitating social environment. Within the environment, the mothers could connect to and reflect on their parenting experiences, which resulted in a level of greater self-development, including the development of their parental-self.

The findings of this study suggest that greater attention should be focused on the supportive function of the treatment environment by a more responsive program approach that will achieve greater integrated treatment outcomes, beyond simply providing "parenting programming." This means a re-examination of the supportive function of the treatment program in a holistic way and a greater application of the relational model as highlighted in previous studies (Byington, 1993; Luthar & Walsh, 1995). Furthermore, this means the application of broader outcome measures as recommended by LaFave and Desporates Echols (1999).

The following supportive elements appeared instrumental in positive treatment outcomes: (1) A parent-child program option that responded to women's desire to continue parenting while in treatment and to come into residential drug treatment with their children. (2) The responsiveness of the program to mothers' social support need that intertwined with their overall expectation of treatment. (3) The considerable support that the child/children's presence provided for the mothers in treatment. (4) The perceived support from various aspects of the treatment, including staff and other mothers, which minimized the adverse effect of the multiple stresses embedded in being in residential drug treatment with their children. (5) The 12- to 18-month timeframe and the residential nature of the program that allowed for a new experience to be formulated–which counteracted the negative, old experiences–and resulted in some level of trust, internalization, and integration of support.

LIMITATION OF THE STUDY

Although the findings generated from the qualitative method can provide valuable direction for future research for similar subject matters, generalization of findings is limited by the small purposeful sampling method employed in this study. Moreover, the data was captured while study participants were still in the program. The findings, therefore, may not be comparable to findings from mothers who have left treatment and are living back in the community. Finally, the findings should not be interpreted within a pure Self-In-Relation model, as all participating programs employed a combined Therapeutic Community Model and a relational approach.

IMPLICATION FOR POLICY, PRACTICE, AND RESEARCH

The qualitative findings, supported by quantitative data, provide valuable directions for policy development, practice examination, and research focus for mothers in drug treatment:

1. *A Mother-Child Program as a Treatment Option Is Critical.* The findings affirm the value of a mother-child residential drug treatment for mothers who desire to continue parenting while in treatment. Hence, providers are strongly recommended to give treatment choice a more central position and more available funding for this type of programming. Furthermore, given that the majority of the mothers perceived that residential drug treatment was their last resort for assuming parenting while receiving treatment, other treatment programs may examine adopting the family-centered and relational-focused approach to serve the mother and child as a unit.

2. *Identifying and Expanding the Supportive Function of the Treatment Program.* More than merely removing treatment barriers, this study identified the significant supportive function that the residential drug treatment program is capable of performing in facilitating a positive parenting experience and shaping a positive parental self. Future research should examine more closely the supportive function of these treatment programs, particularly in the following areas:

- *Individually-Based Therapeutic and Supportive Work.* Individual support provided by the staff regardless of their roles and functions appears imperative in the mothers' development of a rudimentary sense of self and a healthy relationship. Thus, further research is needed to identify how individually-based therapeutic and supportive work can be enhanced.
- *Parenting Programming.* Parenting programming should be further examined to strengthen its goals and functions with particular focus on: (1) individual consultation and support by parenting teachers; (2) programming that engages both the mother and/or her child/ children; (3) parenting classes throughout treatment with topics relevant to the developmental needs of mother and child; and (4) clear policies for working with families of varied composition such as one with older children or with more than one child.

3. *A Higher Level of Integration Between Parenting Programming and Treatment Programming.* The often-changing parenting programming, as reported in this study, suggests that these programs were struggling with its family focus, which undermined the integration of both parenting and substance abuse programmings and compromised the program's provision of support to the mother and child. Greater incorporation of the relational approach and the family-centered approach into programming may minimize this fragmentation and maximize the mothers' gains from treatment. Moreover, the scope of outcome measures should be broadened to address treatment outcomes more integrally and adequately, taking into consideration the different factors in treatment and their interaction in the treatment environment.

4. *Trust Facilitation.* Trust was key in the relationship building with both peer mothers and the staff. Therefore, efforts should be extended to examine ways to deepen the trust between the mothers and staff, including addressing frequent turnover by staff; handling insensitive and/or rigid treatment approaches of the mothers by para-professional staff; encouraging and incorporating mothers' input, particularly concerning parenting, into the programming to ensure and enhance the mothers' partnership with the staff; and investing greater efforts into developing programming to further mother-to-mother support.

CONCLUSION

Parenting is a reality that is faced everyday by mothers in residential drug treatment with their children. It is thus imperative to pay greater attention to how this parenting reality impacts upon the mothers' parenting needs and how these needs can be met more fully during the treatment process. The findings of this study add a piece of much needed information to previous outcome studies that were not mindful of the social support aspect of residential drug treatment and its relation to parenting outcomes.

REFERENCES

Ainsworth, M.D.S. (1968). Object relations, dependency, and attachment: A theoretical review of the infant-mother relationship. *Child Development*, 40, 969-1025.
Belsky, J. (1984). The determinants of parenting: A process model. *Child Devleopment*, 55, 83-96.

Belsky, J., & Vondra, J. (1989). Lessons from child abuse: The determinant of parenting. In D. Cicchetti & V. Carlson (Eds.), *Child maltreatment: Research and theory on the consequence of abuse and neglect* (pp. 153-202). New York: Cambridge University Press.

Benedek, T. (1956). The psychological aspects of parenting. *American Journal of Orthopsychiarty.*

Benedek, T. (1959). Parenthood as a developmental phrase. *Journal of the American Psychoanaytic Association*, 7, 389-417.

Benedek, T. (1970). Motherhood and nurturing. In J.E. Anthony & T. Benedek (Eds.), *Parenthood: Psychology & psychopathology*. Boston: Little, Brown & Co.

Brown, E.R. (1992). Program and staff characteristics in successful treatment. In M.M. Kilbey & K. Ashghar (Eds.), *Methodologies issues in epidemiological, prevention, and treatment research on drug-exposed women and their children* (NIDA Research Monograph No.117, pp. 305-313). Rockville, MD: National Institute on Drug Abuse.

Brown, V.B., Melchoir, L.A., Waite-O'Brien, N., & Huba, G.J (2002). Effects of women-sensitive, long-term residential treatment on psychological functioning of diverse populations of women. *Journal of Substance Abuse Treatment*, 23 (2), 133-144.

Byington, D.B. (1993). *Love and drugs: A relational approach to addiction.* Unpublished manuscript.

Byington, D.B. (1997). Applying relational theory to addiction treatment, in S.L. Straussner and E. Zelvin (Eds.), *Gender and addiction* (pp. 31-46). Northvale, NJ: Jason Aronson.

Camp, J.M., & Finkelstein, N. (1997). Parenting training for women in residential substance abuse treatment: Result of a demonstration project. *Journal of Substance Abuse Treatment*,14.

Carlson, R.G., Siegal, H.A., & Falck, R.S. (1998). Qualitative research methods in drug abuse and AIDS prevention research: An overview. *National Clearinghouse for Alcohol and Drug Information* (Research Monograph 157). Rockville, MD: National Institute on Drug Abuse.

Conners, N.A., Bradley, R.H., Whiteside-Mansell, L., & Crone, C.C. (2001). A comprehensive substance abuse treatment program for women and their children: An initial evaluation. *Journal of Substance Abuse Treatment*, 21(2), 67-75.

Creswell, J.W. (1994). *Research design: Qualitative and quantitative approaches.* Thousand Oaks, CA: Sage.

Daghastani, A. (1988). Psychosocial characteristics of pregnant women. In I.J. Chasnoff (Ed.), *Drugs, alcohol, pregnancy, and parenting* (7-16). Dordrecht, Kluwer Academic Publishers.

Davis, I.P. (1994). Integrating qualitative and quantitative methods in clinical research. In E. Sherman & W.J. Reid (Eds.), *Qualitative research in social work*. New York: Columbia University Press.

Davis, S.K. (1990). Chemical dependency in women: A description of its effects and outcome on adequacy parenting. *Journal of Substance Abuse Treatment*, 7, 225-232.

Demick, J., Bursik, K., & Diabiase, R. (1993). *Parental development*. Hillside, NJ: Lawrence Erlbaum.

Dunst, C.J., Jenkins, V., & Trivette, C.M. (1984). Family Support Scale. In C.J. Dunst; C. Trivette; & A. Deal (Eds.) (1994). *Support and strengthening families: Methods, strategies, & outcomes.* Cambridge, MA: Brookline Books.

Dunst, C.J., & Trivette, C.M. (1988). A family systems model in early intervention with handicapped and developmentally at-risk children. In D. Powell (Ed.), *Parent education as early childhood intervention: Emerging directions in theory, research, and practice* (pp. 131- 179). Norwood, NJ: Ablex.

Dunst, C.J., Trivette, C.M., & Thompson, R. (1990). Supporting and strengthening family functioning: Toward a congruence between principles and practices. *Prevention in Human Services,* 9(1), 19-43.

Ely, M., Anzul, M., Friedman, T., Garner, D., & Steinmetz, A.M. (1991). *Doing qualitative research: Circles within circles.* London: Falmer.

Finkelstein, N. (1993). The relational model. In D. Kronstadt, P.F. Green, & C. Marcus (Eds.), *Pregnancy and exposure to alcohol and other drug use* (Center for Substance Abuse Prevention Technical Bulletin, 7, 45-59). Rockville, MD: U.S. Dept. of Health and Human Services.

Finkelstein, N. (1994). Treatment issues for alcohol- and drug-dependent pregnant and parenting women. *Health and Social Work,* 19, 7-5.

Goldberg, M.E. (1995). Substance-abusing women: False stereotypes and real needs. *Social Work,* 40, 789-798.

Goldberg, M.E., Lex, B.W., Mello, N.K., Mendelson, J.H, Tommie, A., & Bower, M.A. (1996). Impact of maternal alcoholism on separation of children from their mothers: Findings from a sample of incarcerated women. *American Journal of Orthopsychiarty,* 66(2), 228-238.

Gottlieb, B.H. (Ed.). (1981). *Social networks and social support.* Beverly Hills, CA: Sage.

Gottlieb, B.H. (1983). *Social support strategies.* Newbury Park, CA: Sage.

Greenleaf, V.D. (1989). *Women and cocaine.* Chicago: Lowell House.

LaFave, L.M., & Desportes Echols, L. (1999). An argument for choice. An alternative women's treatment program. *Journal of Substance Abuse Treatment,* 16(4), 345-352.

Lincoln, Y.S., & Guba, E.G. (1985). *Naturalistic inquiry.* Beverly Hills, CA: Sage.

Luthar, S.S., & Walsh, K.G. (1995). Treatment needs of drug-addicted mothers: Integrated parenting psychotherapy intervention. *Journal of Substance Abuse Treatment,* 12(5), 341-348.

Mayes, L.C. (1995). Substance abuse and parenting. In M.C. Bornstein (Ed.) et al. *Handbook of parenting, 4: Applied and practical parenting* (pp. 101-125). Mahwah, NJ: Lawrence Erlbaum.

Oakley, A (1992). *Social support & motherhood.* London: Blackwell.

Padgett, D.K. (1998). *Qualitative methods in social work research: Challenges and rewards.* Thousand Oaks, CA: Sage.

Reid, W.J., & Smith, A.D. (1989). *Research in social work* (2nd ed.). New York: Columbia University Press.

Seidman, I. (1998). *Interviewing as qualitative research.* New York: Teachers College Press.

Smyth, N.J., & Miller, B.A. (1997). Parenting issues for substance-abusing women. In S.L. Straussner and E. Zelvin (Eds.), *Gender and addiction* (pp. 123-149). Northvale, NJ: Jason Aronson.

Strass, A., & Corbin, J. (1990). *Basics of qualitative research: Grounded theory procedures and techniques.* Newbury Park, CA: Sage.

Sterk-Elifson, C. (1998). Determining drug use patterns among women: The value of qualitative research methods. *National Clearinghouse of Alcohol and Drug Information* (Research Monograph 157; chapter 4). Rockville, MD: National Institute on Drug Abuse.

Taylor, A. (1993). *Women drug users.* New York: Oxford University Press.

Times, F.M., Jainchill, N., & De Leon, G. (1994). *Therapeutic community and treatment research,* 144,1-15.

Uziel-Miller, N.D., Lyons, J.S., Kissiel, C., & Love, S. (1998). Treatment needs and initial outcomes of a residential recovery program for African-American women and their children. *American Journal on Addictions,* 7(1), 43-50.

VanBremen, J. R., & Chasnoff, I.J. (1994). Policy issues for integrating parenting interventions and addiction treatment for women. *Topics in Early Childhood Special Education, 14*(2), 254-274.

Wells, D.V.B., & Jackson, J.F. (1992). HIV and chemically dependent women: Recommendations for appropriate health care and drug treatment services. *International Journal of Addictions,* 27, 571-585.

Winnicott, D.W. (1965). *The maturational process and the facilitating environment.* NY: International University Press.

Winnicott, D.W. (1971). *Playing and reality.* Middlesex, England: Penguin.

Winnicott, D.W. (1987). The contribution of psychoanalysis to midwifery. In C. Winnicott, R. Shepherd, & M. Davis (Eds.), *Babies and their mothers* (pp.69-89). Reading, MA: Addison-Wesley.

Yaffe, J., Jenson, J.M., & Howard, M.O. (1995). Women and substance abuse: Implications for treatment. *Alcoholism Treatment Quarterly,* 13(2), 1-15.

Zelvin, E. (1997). Codependency issues of substance-abusing women. In S.L. Straussner and E. Zelvin (Eds.), *Gender and addiction* (pp. 47-68). Northvale, NJ: Jason Aronson.

Identifying Children's Needs
When Parents Access Drug Treatment:
The Utility of a Brief Screening Measure

Stefan M. Gruenert
Samantha S. Ratnam
Menka Tsantefski

SUMMARY. This study evaluated whether a brief screening measure of child psychosocial functioning completed by parents could assist drug and alcohol workers to identify which of their client's children needed follow-up support. As part of a broader research and intervention program for 4-13 year old children with substance dependent parents, the Strengths and Difficulties Questionnaire (SDQ) and a broader clinical assessment were completed with the families of 48 children. Validating its usefulness in this population, significant and moderate correlations were found between SDQ scores and workers' assess-

---

Stefan M. Gruenert, DPsych, Dip AOD, was Project Manager for the Nobody's Clients Project, Odyssey Institute of Studies, 211 Victoria Parade, Collingwood Victoria, 3066, Australia (E-mail: sgruenert@odyssey.org.au). Samantha S. Ratnam, BA/BSW, Dip AOD, and Menka Tsantefski, PhD, Dip Ed, were project workers.

This research formed part of the Nobody's Clients Project supported by a grant from the R.E. Ross Trust, Melbourne, Australia and conducted in collaboration with Odyssey House Victoria; The Windana Society; The Salvation Army (Bridge Program); and Newton's Pharmacy, Kensington, all located in Victoria, Australia.

[Haworth co-indexing entry note]: "Identifying Children's Needs When Parents Access Drug Treatment: The Utility of a Brief Screening Measure." Gruenert, Stefan M., Samantha S. Ratnam, and Menka Tsantefski. Co-published simultaneously in *Journal of Social Work Practice in the Addictions* (The Haworth Press, Inc.) Vol. 6, No. 1/2, 2006, pp. 139-154; and: *Impact of Substance Abuse on Children and Families: Research and Practice Implications* (ed: Shulamith Lala Ashenberg Straussner, and Christine Huff Fewell) The Haworth Press, Inc., 2006, pp. 139-154. Single or multiple copies of this article are available for a fee from The Haworth Document Delivery Service [1-800-HAWORTH, 9:00 a.m. - 5:00 p.m. (EST). E-mail address: docdelivery@haworthpress.com].

Available online at http://www.haworthpress.com/web/JSWPA
doi:10.1300/J160v06n01_07

ments of children's social, emotional, and cognitive development and schooling. *[Article copies available for a fee from The Haworth Document Delivery Service: 1-800-HAWORTH. E-mail address: <docdelivery@ haworthpress.com> Website: <http://www.HaworthPress.com> © 2006 by The Haworth Press, Inc. All rights reserved.]*

KEYWORDS: Strengths and Difficulties Questionnaire (SDQ), validity, children, screening, families, drug and alcohol treatment

INTRODUCTION

Parental drug use can seriously harm children from conception through adulthood (ACMD, 2003). Drug use during pregnancy has been associated with poor fetal growth and development, the contraction of viral infections, fetal alcohol spectrum disorders and infant withdrawal following birth (Hogan, 1998; Kaltenbach, 1994; Klee, Jackson, & Lewis, 2002). However, the harm of parental drug use more commonly arises from environmental causes such as inadequate physical care, abuse, anti-social role modelling, and compromised parenting (Dunn, Tarter, Mezzich, Vanyukov, Kirisci, & Kirillova, 2002; Gruenert, Ratnam, & Tsantefski, 2004).

The problematic use of alcohol or other drugs by parents has been identified as a major risk factor for children's early-onset substance use in several longitudinal studies (Kaplow, Curran, & Dodge, 2002). In addition, the children of alcohol and drug dependent parents have an elevated risk of developing their own substance abuse problems due to the presence of genetic, biological, and family environmental factors (Kumpfer, 1999).

While it should not be assumed that parental drug use necessarily leads to negative outcomes for all children, those raised by one or more substance dependent parents are likely to live in relative poverty, experience school failure, and develop a range of emotional and behavioural problems (Dawe, Harnett, Rendalls, & Staiger, 2003; Patton, 2003). Such children are also at increased risk of emotional and physical neglect and abuse. Consequently, a large proportion of families referred to child protection services in Australia (DHS, 2002) and elsewhere (Nair et al., 1997) involve some degree of problematic parental drug or alcohol use.

Research demonstrates that outcomes are better the earlier prevention programs reach children (Kumpfer, 1999; Luthar, Cushing, Merikangas, & Rounsaville, 1998). In view of this, focus on the early detection and treatment of emotional adjustment or behavioural problems in children appears warranted. However, children with alcohol and drug dependent parents can be difficult to access. Many parents with drug or alcohol problems do not seek help from community child and family services because they fear the removal of their children by welfare authorities.

Drug treatment services often have privileged access to this population when they are most motivated to make changes to address the needs of their whole family. Unfortunately, few drug and alcohol workers have the skills or time available to conduct broad assessments of their clients' children, or to visit families in their homes. Consequently, many at risk children go undetected until extreme child protective issues surface or children's own mental health problems or behaviors escalate and an opportunity for targeted early intervention is missed. A screening measure of children's psychosocial functioning is therefore needed to assist drug treatment clinicians to identify children's problems as early as possible.

To be useful during assessment, the screening measure ought to be brief, cost effective, simple to use, reliable, and valid within this population. Such a tool would enhance the decision making of drug and alcohol workers by helping them to identify those families requiring follow-up assessment, support, or referrals without requiring them to assess children directly or have a great deal of knowledge about children's psychological well-being.

THE STRENGTHS AND DIFFICULTIES QUESTIONNAIRE (SDQ)

Goodman (1997) has recently developed a child psycho-social screening measure, the Strengths and Difficulties Questionnaire (SDQ), which is gaining recognition in the UK, Europe, and Australia as a research and clinical screening tool (Mellor, 2004). Self-report, teacher completed, and parent completed versions of the measure each take about five minutes to administer. The measure contains five subscales assessing emotional symptoms, conduct problems, hyperactivity-inattention, peer problems, and pro-social behavior.

Currently, the measure can be obtained without charge and has demonstrated reliability and validity within clinical and community populations in Europe (e.g., Muris, Meesters, & van den Berg, 2003; Goodman, 2001; Goodman, Renfrew, & Mullick, 2000) and in Australia (Mathai, Anderson, & Bourne, 2002). Strong correlations have been found between the self-report, teacher-report, and parent report version indicating high inter-informant reliability (Goodman, 1997, 2001; Goodman, Ford, Simmons, Gatward, & Meltzer, 2003; Muris et al., 2003). For example, in a recent Australian community sample of over 900 children aged between 7 and 17 years, internal reliability coefficients of the sub-scales and total difficulties score ranged from .67 to .80 for the parent version; the test-retest reliability of the parent version was .81 for the total difficulties score at a two-week follow-up, while the parent-teacher, parent-child, and teacher-child inter-informant correlations of the total difficulties score were .46, .45, and .45 respectively (Mellor, 2004).

The original SDQ was validated against Rutter questionnaires (Goodman, 1997), with the SDQ being comparable to or outperforming the Rutter questionnaires on ability to distinguish psychiatric and dental clinic attendees, inter-informant reliability, brevity, and better coverage of inattention, peer relationships and pro-social behaviour. Later research also suggested that the SDQ is comparable to, or better than, the widely used but expensive Achenbach's Child Behaviour Checklist (CBCL) in detecting childhood disorders diagnosed through standardized clinical assessments (Goodman & Scott, 1999; Klasen et al, 2000). In a study of 132 children aged 4-7 years, Goodman and Scott (1999) found CBCL and SDQ scores to be highly correlated and equally able to discriminate psychiatric from dental clients. The SDQ was also significantly better than the CBCL at detecting inattention and hyperactivity, and at least as good at detecting internalizing and externalizing problems when judged against a semi-structured clinical interview. In addition, mothers of low-risk children were twice as likely to prefer the SDQ. Likewise, Klasen and colleagues (2000) found similar results in their sample of 273 children drawn from psychiatric clinics (N = 163) and from a community sample (N = 110) in Germany.

In a recent Australian study of 130 children, a computerized algorithm predicted child psychiatric diagnoses based on the parent, teacher, and self-report SDQ scores within a child and adolescent mental health service (Mathai, Anderson, & Bourne, 2003). The level of agreement between the SDQ generated diagnoses and the diagnoses of a multidisciplinary community outpatient team was moderate to high (ranging from 0.39 to 0.56) and was also moderate for an independent clinician who examined the case notes and was blind to SDQ scores (ranging from 0.26 to 0.43). All correlations were significant.

The reported sensitivity of the measure in detecting conduct-oppositional disorders, hyperactivity disorders, depression, pervasive developmental disorders, and some anxiety disorders in community and clinical samples ranges between 70% and 90% and between 30% and 50% for other anxiety disorders and eating disorders (Goodman et al., 2003; Goodman, Renfrew, & Mullick, 2000).

The validity of the parent completed version of the SDQ as a screening measure has not been assessed with substance dependent parents regarding their children. The validity of the SDQ in this population is of special interest. The illicit nature and stigma of parental drug dependencies and the associated fear of child removal by welfare authorities has lead to the assumption that parental reports cannot be trusted and that broad psychosocial assessments in the home environment, completed by trained staff, are required for the early detection of children's problems.

This study therefore aimed to assess the usefulness and validity of the SDQ as a screening measure of child psychosocial functioning when parents accessed treatment for their drug or alcohol problems, by comparing the parent version SDQ scores with clinical child and family assessments completed by project workers.

METHOD

The 'Nobody's Clients' Project

This study was conducted as part of a larger research, which targeted a prevention and early intervention program for 4-13 year old children with substance dependent parents. Children participating in the 'Nobody's Clients' project had at least one parent receiving drug treatment from a residential rehabilitation, outpatient counseling, supported accommodation, or pharmacotherapy program in Melbourne, Australia. The project aimed to identify and then address the needs of these children. Children in this age range were chosen because research and intervention programs catering for both younger as well as older children seemed to be more prevalent in Australia.

Intensive short-term case management was provided to children for a minimum of three months while their experiences were documented.

The total time spent with each child and their family members ranged from five to 36 hours (M = 12 hours). Most family contact occurred in the children's or other family members' homes. Some contact occurred in drug treatment facilities or in a recreational context.

Following the assessment period and the establishment of a therapeutic alliance, feedback was provided to caregivers about family strengths and areas of concern, especially those in which children's needs were not being addressed. Goals were then set in collaboration with family members to address these concerns, to reduce risk factors, to strengthen protective factors, and to improve family functioning.

Problems experienced by children included: neglect; physical, verbal, and sexual abuse; grief and trauma related to parental overdose and death; general anxiety and phobias; social isolation; "parentified" behaviours; conduct problems such as aggression, biting, and inappropriate sexual displays; and a lack of opportunities for recreation and play.

In response to identified needs, project workers provided individual and family counselling to children and other family members as well as other services including helping parents: develop parenting skills; improve household routines and budgets; developed plans for children's care in the event of parent relapse; resolve family conflicts; strengthen the communication and relationships with children's schools and other community networks; and remove barriers so as to improve school attendance rates. Many children were also enrolled in recreational activities such as sports, school holiday programs, and camps. When longer-term or specialist support was required, referrals were made to other community-based agencies such as mentoring, specialist education, or mental health services. [Further information about the project can be found in the full report by Gruenert, Ratnam, & Tsantefski (2004).]

Participants

Children. Forty-eight children (56% male) along with 72 members of their families participated on a voluntary basis in the Nobody's Clients Project. Children ranged in age from four to 13 years, with a mean age of 7.4 years (*SD* = 2.6). Eighty-eight percent of children were of Australian (Anglo-Celtic) decent, 8% of children were of Australian Aboriginal decent, and 4% had other ethnic backgrounds.

Parents. Parents receiving drug or alcohol treatment were aged between 22 and 48 years with a mean age of 32.4 years (*SD* = 5.6). Fifty-six percent were the child's biological mother, 42% their biological father and 6% a stepparent, including 4% with both biological parents in treatment. Most were polydrug users with a long history of substance dependency. The most problematic drug was heroin for 38% of parents, alcohol (27%), and cannabis (17%), with 18% of parents preferring another drug (mostly amphetamines). About 70% of parents had been previously charged with at least one criminal offence.

Caregivers. During the assessment period, children were being cared for by single biological mothers (44%), single biological fathers (21%), grandparents (19%), one biological parent and their partner (6%), another relative (8%), or were in foster care (2%). For some children, contact with their parent receiving treatment had been irregular. In many cases (63%), the parent receiving treatment had also been the person most responsible for raising the child. For a few children (10%), primary care givers were biological parents who had also experienced problematic substance use but were not currently receiving treatment. For others (27%), children's primary care givers were parents, relatives, or foster carers with no history of drug treatment.

Measures

All measures, including demographic information, clinical assessment questions, and summary assessment domains were contained in a 50-page, semi-structured interview.

Strengths and Difficulties Questionnaire. The parent version of the Strengths and Difficulties Questionnaire (SDQ), a brief behavioural screening tool of 4 to 16 year old children (Goodman, 1997), was used to assess children's functioning. The scale consists of 25 items, 10 of which are statements of strengths (e.g., thinks things out before acting), 14 which are statements of difficulty (e.g., many fears, easily scared), and one which is neutral (e.g., gets on better with adults than with other children). Responses are scored on a three-point scale, 0–"not true," 1–"somewhat true," or 2–"certainly true." Five clinical scales, each of consisting of 5-items (emotional symptoms, conduct problems, hyperactivity-inattention, peer problems, and pro-social or positive behaviors) can be derived, ranging in score from 0 to 10. A total problem score ranging from 0 to 40 is calculated by summing all scales except the pro-social scale.

An additional supplement also records information on chronicity, distress, social impairment, and the burden on others of the child's problems. The various versions, associated papers, and norms based on British, American, Finish, German, and Swedish data differentiating normal, borderline, and abnormal scores can be found at *www.sdqinfo.com*.

Australian norms for children aged 7 years to 17 years have recently been produced (Mellor, 2005). These were based on a representative community sample of 910 children, their parents and their teachers, randomly drawn from 100 schools across the State of Victoria. Australian cut-off scores distinguishing normal, borderline, and abnormal adjustment were found to vary between gender, age, and informant versions, and across subscales and the total difficulties score. Cut-off scores were derived in the same way as the original UK version, based on the supposition that about 10% of children in the community have a significant mental health problem, and a further 10% have a borderline problem. The borderline classification is therefore given to scores between the 80th and 89th percentile, and the abnormal classification given to scores beyond the 90th percentile. Mellor (2005) suggests, however, that because the tool is primarily used as a screening and evaluation tool, rather than a diagnostic measure, terms such as "borderline" and "abnormal" should be avoided with preference for terms such as "query" and "of-concern." This also reflects the fact that cut-off scores were not based on actual diagnosed problems of children in the sample used to create the norms.

Child and Family Assessment (CFA). The Child and Family Assessment was specifically developed by the authors for the purpose of this study. It was based on a literature review of suggested outcome domains to measure when evaluating interventions for children with substance dependent parents (Kumpfer, 1999), and the risk and protective factors relating to children with substance dependent parents (Aldridge, 1999; Davis & Owen, 1999; Hawkins, Catalano, & Miller, 1992; Zucker & Fitzgerald, 1991). Factors identified from this literature were summarized into ten domains, five relating to the child: Biological & Health, Schooling & Cognitive Development, Emotional & Behavioural Development, Social Development, and Drug Exposure & Criminal Environment, and five relating to the broader family: Physical Environment, Parenting, Family Functioning, Social Support, and Parent-Child Attachment. Notable omissions were genetic factors, peer norms about drug use (due to the age of children involved), and children's temperament.

Content areas that were assessed within each of these ten domains are summarized in the Appendix. A summary rating ranging between 1 and 7 was made by project workers for each area of content. An average score for each domain was then calculated. A score of 1 indicates severe problems and low functioning, while a score of 7 indicates few or no problems and high functioning.

The three authors, who also conducted the assessments and interventions, were social work and psychology trained clinicians with between one and ten years experience in working with substance dependent parents and their children. In order to maximize the agreement between different informant ratings on the CFA, a number of case studies were examined and independently rated by the authors prior to any project work. Any disagreements (defined as a difference of more than 1-point on the summary scores) were discussed until consensus about the interpretation and scoring was reached.

Procedure

Families were recruited from four different drug treatment agencies in the city of Melbourne, Australia. Within these participating agencies, brochures advertising the project were given to clients who were parents of at least one child in the age range. Once consent had been obtained from the parent receiving treatment and from other caregivers, the children and their families were assessed using the semi-structured interview. Drawings and play were also used to build rapport with children and to help them to tell stories about their experiences within their families. When appropriate, written reports were examined and school or kindergarten teachers and any other workers were consulted. Assessments and interviews took place over multiple home or treatment facility visits, and generally required between 3 and 6 hours to complete.

RESULTS

Average scores on the sub-domains of the SDQ completed by primary care givers indicated that children had significantly greater Emotional symptoms, Conduct problems, Hyperactivity, and Peer problems than children in the general Australian community, but had no worse Pro-Social behaviours (see Table 1).

Although the level of psychosocial functioning of children who participated in the project was lower than Australian children on average, there was a great deal of diversity in the sample. Based on their SDQ total difficulty scores and the Australian normative data, each child was coded as being "of concern" if they fell within the abnormal range for their age and gender, coded as a "query" if they fell within the borderline range for their age and gender, or coded as "normal" if their scores were below these val-

TABLE 1. Sample and Population Means, Standard Deviations, and Internal Reliability Coefficients for the Parent Version of the SDQ

	SDQ Scale	Emotional Symptoms	Conduct problems	Hyper-activity	Peer problems	Pro-social	Total Difficulties score
Parent Completed Version	Possible Range	0-10	0-10	0-10	0-10	0-10	0-40
Total Australian Population	*M* SD	2.1 2.0	1.5 1.6	3.1 2.4	1.6 1.9	8.3 1.7	8.2 6.1
Study Sample	*M* SD	3.6** 2.6	3.0** 2.4	4.3** 2.4	2.3* 2.0	7.8[ns] 1.7	13.2** 6.5
N = 48	α	.71	.72	.74	.62	.62	.82

Note: Differences from population mean **$p < .001$, *$p < .01$, [ns]-not significant at $p > .01$ (one-tail)

ues. No norms exist for children younger than seven years, hence the cut off values for 7-10 year old children were used for children aged 4 to 7 years. An examination of normative data for younger children in other countries suggests that this was an acceptable, albeit a somewhat conservative strategy. The diversity and extent of children's problems in the sample is highlighted in Figure 1. Fifty-six percent of children were classified as "normal," 20 percent scored in the borderline range and were classified as "query," while 24 percent scored in the abnormal range and were classified as "of concern."

As Australian norms differed by age and gender, partial correlations controlling for age and gender were used to evaluate the validity of the SDQ. Partial correlations were calculated between parent-rated total SDQ scores and worker ratings on the 10 domains of the CFA. Due to the large number of correlations calculated and the expected direction of associations, significance was tested at the $\alpha = 0.01$ level (one-tailed).

As shown in Table 2, moderately significant negative correlations were found between worker ratings of Schooling & Cognitive Development, Emotional & Behavioural Development, and Social Development domains of the CFA and the parent-rated SQD Total Difficulties score. No other significant associations were found between the CFA domains and the SDQ total score. As shown in Table 2, several significant correlations were also found between the SDQ sub-domains and the domains of the CFA.

FIGURE 1. Children's SDQ Total Difficulties Scores Compared with Australian Norms

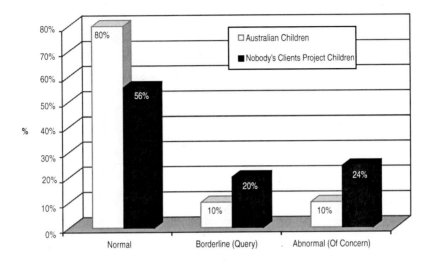

TABLE 2. Partial Correlations Between Worker-Rated Child and Family Domains and Parent-Rated SDQ Total Difficulties and Sub-Domain Scores, Controlling for Children's Age and Gender

	SDQ					
	Total Score	Emotional	Conduct	Hyper-activity	Peers	Pro-social
Child Domains						
Biological & Health	−.31	−.39*	−.06	−.05	−.40**	.06
Schooling & Cognitive Development	−.37*	−.29	−.06	−.40**	−.27	−.10
Emotional & Behavioral Development	−.45**	−.40**	−.33	−.18	−.37*	.02
Social Development	−.46**	−.37	−.34	−.14	−.48**	.11
Drug Exposure & Criminal Environment	.16	.00	.26	.13	.06	−.02
Family Domains						
Physical Environment	−.20	−.15	−.15	−.08	−.20	−.10
Parenting	−.26	−.34	−.21	−.02	−.17	−.18
Family Functioning	−.19	−.37*	−.08	.16	−.25	−.01
Social Support	−.28	−.43**	−.09	.06	−.34	−.02
Parent-Child Attachment	−.28	−.44**	−.15	−.03	−.13	−.09

Note: **p < .005 (one-tail), *p < .01 (one-tail), all other correlations not significant (p > .001, one-tail)

DISCUSSION

Consistent with previous findings in other Australian settings (Mathai, Anderson, & Bourne, 2002), the SDQ was found to be a useful screening measure of child psycho-social functioning when used with parents accessing treatment for their substance dependencies. The SDQ demonstrated adequate internal reliability in this population and worker ratings of a child's cognitive development and schooling, their emotional and behavioural development, and their social development on the CFA were significantly and moderately related to their parent-rated SDQ total difficulties scores. Moreover, associations between parent-rated SDQ total score and other CFA domains were weaker and non-significant.

An examination of the correlations between parent-rated SDQ subscales and the domains of the CFA also reveal a pattern consistent with high external validity of the SDQ. In particular, the emotional symptoms sub-scale of the SDQ was associated with the emotional and behavioural development domain of the CFA, the hyperactivity-inattention sub-scale of the SDQ was associated with the schooling and cognitive development domain of the CFA and the peer problems sub-scale of the SDQ was associated with the social development domain of the CFA. Other associations suggest that peer problems identified by the SDQ were also related to children's health, physical appearance, and physical development identified by the CFA, and that emotional symptoms identified by the SDQ were related to the level of support that children and parents received, their level of housing stability, and parent-child attachment as identified by the CFA.

Limitations of Study

Several issues necessitate caution in generalizing these findings to the larger population of children with substance dependent parents until these results can be replicated in other samples. The small sample size and the lack of standardised data about the clinical assessment used are clear limitations of this study. While project workers were involved in the development and interpretation of the CFA used in this study, no inter-rater reliability measures were recorded when used with sample participants. In addition, Australian SDQ norms do not currently exist for children younger than seven years of age, which accounts for approximately 46% of this sample. However, given that the analysis controlled for age and gender affects and relied on associations between

SDQ total scores and not the normative cut-offs, the lack of normative data for younger children was less problematic. Furthermore, the psychometric properties of the SDQ have been well established in numerous other contexts.

CONCLUSION

These findings indicate that the quick and cost effective SDQ provides an effective and valid way of screening for children's problems when used at assessment with parents accessing drug treatment. In the absence of trained staff with the resources to conduct full clinical assessments on children, the SDQ provides an alternative approach to identifying children in need of support.

Interventions with children identified as having social and behavioral problems will depend on worker knowledge, training, and service flexibility. Where possible, further assessment questions about any traumatic events that the child has been exposed to should be also asked. Family routines, stability, functioning, and current external support could also be examined. If staff resources are available, similar interventions to those used in the Nobody's Clients project may ensure that the safety of children is maintained while parents access drug treatment and assist children to feel more in control within their home environment, strengthen their commitment to school and trust in family members, help develop their social skills, and rebuild self-esteem and self-efficacy. Alternatively, referrals could be made to other existing community based agencies that offer such child and family support.

When introducing screening for children's well-being in settings where the adult is the primary client, it will be important to ensure that staff feel adequately trained and supervised to respond to any child problems that they may identify, whether directly or through referrals. Staff members may also be concerned about maintaining their client's trust while enquiring about children's well-being, and the consequences for the therapeutic alliance if a notification to child protection authorities becomes necessary. Notwithstanding these difficulties, the SDQ offers significant benefits for early intervention in at-risk children when used as a screening measure in adult drug treatment services.

Future research should examine the types of problems present in children who are classified as "abnormal" or "of-concern" by the SDQ. Research should also examine ways of identifying at-risk infants and younger children of substance dependent parents as these are often the children at most risk. The extent to which drug and alcohol agencies actually assess and then respond to the needs of their clients' children also needs to be monitored, as does the long-term effectiveness of any targeted intervention programs that are developed and delivered to families with substance dependent parents.

REFERENCES

ACMD (2003). *Hidden harm: Responding to the needs of children of problem drug users*. Advisory Council on the Misuse of Drugs, Home Office: UK.

Aldridge, T. (1999). Rethinking children's needs living with drug-using parents, *Family Values* (March/April), 8-11.

Davis, C., & Owen, L. (1999). *Action research evaluation of the Odyssey House Family Program* (Final Report). Victoria: Department of Social Work and Social Policy, LaTrobe University, Australia.

Dawe, S., Harnett, P.H., Rendalls, V., & Staiger, P. (2003). Improving family functioning and child outcome in methadone maintained families: The Parents Under Pressure programme. *Drug and Alcohol Review, 22*, 299-307.

DHS (2002). *Protocol between drug treatment services and child protection for working with parents with alcohol and other drug issues*. community Care Division, Department of Human Services, Victoria, Australia.

Dunn, M. G., Tarter, R. E., Mezzich, A. C., Vanyukov, M., Kirisci, L., & Kirillova, G. (2002). Origins and consequences of child neglect in substance abuse families. *Clinical Psychology Review, 22*(7), 1063-90.

Goodman R. (1997). The Strengths and Difficulties questionnaire: A research note. *Journal of Child Psychology & Psychiatry, 38*, 581-586.

Goodman R. (2001). Psychometric properties of the Strengths and Difficulties Questionnaire. *Journal of the American Academy of Child & Adolescent Psychiatry, 40*, 1337-1345.

Goodman, R., Renfrew, D., & Mullick, M. (2000). Predicting type of psychiatric disorder from Strengths and Difficulties Questionnaire (SDQ) scores in child mental health clinics in London and Dhaka. *European Child and Adolescent Psychiatry, 9*,129-134.

Goodman, R., Ford, T., Simmons, H., Gatward, R., & Meltzer, H. (2003). Using the Strengths and Difficulties Questionnaire (SDQ) to screen for child psychiatric disorders in a community sample. *International Review of Psychiatry, 15*, 166-172.

Goodman, R., & Scott, S. (1999). Comparing the Strengths and Difficulties Questionnaire and the Child Behaviour Checklist: Is small beautiful? *Journal of Abnormal Child Psychology, 27*(1), 17-24.

Gruenert, S.M., Ratnam, S.S., & Tsantefski, M. (2004). *The Nobody's Clients Project: Full Report*. Odyssey Institute of Studies, Odyssey House Victoria: Australia. (available for download at *www.odyssey.org.au*).

Hawkins, J. D., Catalano, R.F., & Miller, J.Y. (1992). Risk and protective factors for alcohol and other drug problems in adolescence and early adulthood: Implications for substance abuse prevention. *Psychological Bulletin, 112*(1), 64-105.

Hogan, D. M. (1998). Annotation: The psychological development and welfare of children of opiate and cocaine users: Review and research needs. *Journal of Child Psychology & Psychiatry, 39*(5), 609-620.

Kaltenbach, K. (1994). Effects of in-utero opiate exposure: New paradigms for old questions. *Drug and Alcohol Dependencies, 36*, 83-87.

Kaplow, J. B., Curran, P. J., & Dodge, K. A. (2002). Child, parent, and peer predictors of early-onset substance use: A multi-site longitudinal study. *Journal of Abnormal Child Psychology, 30*(3), 199-216.

Klasen, H., Woerner, W., Wolke, D., Meyer, R., Overmeyer, S., Kaschnitz, W., Rothenberger, A., & Goodman, R. (2000). Comparing the German versions of the Strengths and Difficulties Questionnaire (SDQ-Deu) and the Child Behavior Checklist. *European Child and Adolescent Psychiatry, 9*, 271-276.

Klee, H., Jackson, M., & Lewis, S. (2002). *Drug misuse and motherhood,* Routledge, London.

Kumpfer, K. L. (1999). Outcome Measures of Interventions in the Study of Children of Substance-abusing Parents. *Paediatrics, 103*(5), 1128-1144.

Luthar, S. S., Cushing, G., Merikangas, K.R., & Rounsaville, B.J. (1998). Multiple jeopardy: Risk and protective factors among addicted mothers' offspring. *Development and Psychopathology, 10*, 117-136.

Mathai, J., Anderson, P., & Bourne, A. (2002). The Strengths and Difficulties Questionnaire (SDQ) as a screening measure prior to admission to a Child and Adolescent Mental Health Service (CAMHS). *Australian e-Journal for the Advancement of Mental Health (AeJAMH), 1*(3).

Mathai, J., Anderson, P., & Bourne, A. (2003). Use of the Strengths and Difficulties Questionnaire as an outcome measure in a child and adolescent mental health service. *Australian Psychiatry,* 11, 334-337.

Mellor, D. (2004). Furthering the use of the Strengths and Difficulties Questionnaire: Reliability with younger child respondents. *Psychological Assessment,* 16(4), 396-401.

Mellor, D. (2005). *Community Norms for the Strengths and Difficulties Questionnaire in Australia.* School of Psychology, Deakin University, Australia.

Muris, P., Meesters, C., & van den Berg, F. (2003). The Strengths and Difficulties Questionnaire (SDQ): Further evidence for its reliability and validity in a community sample of Dutch children and adolescents. *European Child and Adolescent Psychiatry, 12*, 1-8.

Nair, P., Black, M.M., Schuler, M., Keane, V., Snow, L., Rigney, B.A., & Magder, L. (1997). Risk factors for disruption in primary care giving among infants of substance abusing women. *Child Abuse & Neglect, 21,* 1039-1051.

Patton, N. (2003). *Parental drug use–The bigger picture: A review of the literature.* The Mirabel Foundation: Melbourne, Australia.

Zucker, R. A., & Fitzgerald, H. E. (1991). Early developmental factors and risk for alcohol problems. *Alcohol Health & Research World, 15,* 1-24.

APPENDIX

Domains and Content of the Worker-Rated Child and Family Assessment

The Child	The Family
• Biological & Health 　□ Physical appearance 　□ Hospital admissions 　□ Sickness & visits to the doctor 　□ Age appropriate physical development 　□ Age appropriate motor skills 　□ Documented effects of in-utero exposure to drugs	• Physical Environment 　□ Adequate food, clothing, and shelter 　□ Appropriate mental stimulus for child in family/home environment 　□ Safety/supervision in child's home environment
• Schooling & Cognitive Development 　□ School attendance 　□ Attentiveness in class 　□ Academic performance 　□ Attitude to learning (motivation) 　□ Completion of homework 　□ Participation in extra-curricular activities 　□ Language or learning difficulties	• Parenting 　□ Knowledge of child development 　□ Availability and attentiveness to child 　□ Practical parenting skills 　□ Self-esteem/efficacy in parenting ability 　□ Self-care activities 　□ Values/beliefs/attitudes to parenting 　□ Emotional support for child
• Emotional & Behaviourial Development 　□ Overall mood 　□ Rage of affects 　□ Depth and appropriateness of affect 　□ Anxiety and fear 　□ Anger or aggressive outbursts 　□ Self-esteem/self-concept/Identity	• Family Functioning 　□ Ability to solve problems/conflicts 　□ Communication between family members 　□ Appropriateness of roles assumed by/imposed on family members 　□ Engagement in family activities 　□ Intensity and frequency of conflict 　□ Family togetherness/team work
• Social Development 　□ Age appropriate dialogue 　□ Interaction with other children/peers 　□ Interaction with adults 　□ Problem behaviors/temperament 　□ Responsive to environment 　□ Liked by peers	• Social Support 　□ Child's access to friends or supportive adults 　□ Child's access to formal social support 　□ Caregiver's access to friends or supportive adults 　□ Caregiver's access to formal social support 　□ Family stability/house moves/long-term friends
• Drug Exposure & Criminal Environment 　□ Exposure to caregiver's drug taking 　□ Exposure to criminal activities 　□ Access to other role models 　□ Child's use of drugs/alcohol 　□ Child's involvement in criminal activity 　□ Drug/crime saturated residential area	• Attachment 　□ Displays of affection or closeness 　□ Child's confidence to explore/interact with others 　□ Behaviour control/discipline of child 　□ Caregiver-child interactions 　□ Caregiver's care and concern for child

Adolescents in Treatment: Effects of Parental Substance Abuse on Treatment Entry Characteristics and Outcomes

Gillian Leichtling
Roy M. Gabriel
Chandra K. Lewis
Kelly Jean Vander Ley

SUMMARY. Research strongly supports an increased risk of substance use disorders among the adolescent children of addicted parents. However, little documentation exists of how these adolescents fare when they present for treatment. This article uses data taken from a two-state study

Gillian Leichtling, BA, is Research Associate (E-mail: gillian_leichtling@rmccorp.com), Roy M. Gabriel, PhD, is Senior Research Associate (E-mail: roy_gabriel@rmccorp.com), Chandra K. Lewis, MA, is Research Assistant (E-mail: chandra_lewis@rmccorp. com), and Kelly Jean Vander Ley, PhD, is Senior Research Associate (E-mail: kelly_vanderley@rmccorp.com), all with the RMC Research Corporation, 552 SW Fifth Avenue, Suite 1407, Portland, OR 97204-2131.

Funding for this study was provided by the Substance Abuse and Mental Health Services Administration (SAMHSA) Center for Substance Abuse Treatment (CSAT) through Cooperative Agreements Tl 11333 and Tl 12045. The authors also gratefully acknowledge the assistance of their colleagues Trey Guy and Kathy Laws.

[Haworth co-indexing entry note]: "Adolescents in Treatment: Effects of Parental Substance Abuse on Treatment Entry Characteristics and Outcomes." Leichtling, Gillian et al. Co-published simultaneously in *Journal of Social Work Practice in the Addictions* (The Haworth Press, Inc.) Vol. 6, No. 1/2, 2006, pp. 155-174; and: *Impact of Substance Abuse on Children and Families: Research and Practice Implications* (ed: Shulamith Lala Ashenberg Straussner, and Christine Huff Fewell) The Haworth Press, Inc., 2006, pp. 155-174. Single or multiple copies of this article are available for a fee from The Haworth Document Delivery Service [1-800-HAWORTH, 9:00 a.m. - 5:00 p.m. (EST). E-mail address: docdelivery@haworthpress.com].

on the effects of adolescent substance abuse treatment to examine the characteristics of adolescents with substance-abusing parents and their outcomes following an episode of outpatient treatment. Although such adolescents enter treatment with greater problem severity in a range of areas, outcomes appear similar to adolescents with no substance-abusing parents. The impact of family and individual counseling on outcomes was also examined, demonstrating mixed results for adolescents with substance-abusing parents. *[Article copies available for a fee from The Haworth Document Delivery Service: 1-800-HAWORTH. E-mail address: <docdelivery@haworthpress.com> Website: <http://www.HaworthPress.com> © 2005 by The Haworth Press, Inc. All rights reserved.]*

KEYWORDS. Adolescent treatment, parental substance abuse, treatment outcomes, family counseling

INTRODUCTION

A large body of literature on children of substance abusers, primarily focused on the children of alcoholics, documents an increased risk of substance use disorders for these children (Anda, Whitfield, Felitti, Chapman, Edwards, Dube et al., 2002; Chassin, Pitts, DeLucia, & Todd, 1999; Johnson & Leff, 1999). Children of alcoholics and other substance abusers may be more likely to experience problems in personal and social functioning, particularly externalizing problems such as aggression, impulsivity, and disruptive behavior disorders (Puttler, Zucker, Fitzgerald, & Bingham, 1998; Sher, 1997). Parental alcoholism has also been linked to adolescent internalizing disorders, such as depression and anxiety (Chassin et al., 1999). Evidence also exists of a greater likelihood of dysfunctional family environments for children of alcoholics, including greater conflict and lower cohesion (Friedman & Utada, 1992; Sher, 1991), and family disruption may be associated with children's psychosocial problems (Menees & Segrin, 2000; Stanger, Kamon, Dumenci, Higgins, Bickel, Brabowski et al., 2002). A growing body of research isolates co-occurring psychological disorders of the parents, specifically antisocial personality disorder, as a causal factor in psychosocial problems of the children of alcoholics (Ellis, Zucker, & Fitzgerald, 1997; Schuckit, Smith, Radziminski, & Heyneman, 2000). Antisocial personality disorder appears to be far more common in abusers of alcohol than in people without alcohol abuse (Zucker, 1994). Among families with parents with co-occurring disorders, a host of risk factors (substance dependence, psychopathology, violence, etc.) may act in concert to foster elevated risk among their children (Ellis, Zucker, & Fitzgerald, 1997).

The majority of research on the children of substance abusers to date has examined the behavioral and psychological characteristics of children of substance-abusers. Treatment technology and outcomes for adolescent children of substance abusers, however, remain largely unexamined. Innovations in adolescent treatment interventions over the years have led to an increased focus on family systems and on addressing the dynamics in the family in which the adolescent resides (Ozechowski & Liddle, 2000). Research has shown positive outcomes for family-centered treatment approaches for adolescent substance-abusers (Coatsworth, Santisteban, McBride, & Szapocznik, 2001; Liddle, Dakof, Parker, Diamond, Barrett, & Tejeda, 2001; Rowe & Liddle, 2003). In light of this, the question arises: does and should treatment for adolescents with substance-abusing parents differ in form, content, or effect from that provided to other adolescents in treatment?

A review of the literature using Internet-based abstract databases reveals a limited amount of research on the effectiveness of family therapy for adolescents with substance-abusing parents; what does exist has focused on prevention or on substance use outcomes for parents in treatment (Catalano, Gainey, Fleming, Haggerty, & Johnson, 1999; Edwards & Steinglass, 1995). In addition, little clinical guidance appears to be available on treatment practices for adolescents whose parents also abuse substances. Center for Substance Abuse Treatment's Treatment Improvement Protocols (TIP) and Technical Assistance Publications (TAP) dealing with adolescent treatment have not yet addressed the issue of parental substance abuse.

At least one widely-available manualized treatment model uses parent education sessions to motivate parents to refrain from using alcohol or other drugs in the presence of their adolescent children (Godley, Meyers, Smith, Karvinen, Titus, Godley, Dent, Passetti, & Kelberg, 2001). Edwards and Steinglass' meta-analysis of family therapy (1995) concludes that family therapy is an effective tool in motivating parents into treatment for alcoholism, and Catalano et al. (1999) found that family therapy yielded positive changes in parents' substance use and parenting skills. Further research is needed examining whether substance abuse interventions for parents may be influential in achieving successful outcomes for adolescents in treatment.

RESEARCH QUESTIONS

To explore the treatment needs and treatment outcomes of adolescents with substance-abusing parents, we examined the following questions:

- Among adolescents presenting for treatment, do children of substance abusers differ from those without substance-abusing parents in life experiences, substance use severity, mental health, and other variables?
- Does the treatment adolescents with substance-abusing parents receive differ from that of their peers, particularly in access to family and individual counseling?
- How do substance use and mental health outcomes for adolescents whose parents are active substance abusers compare to those of other adolescents? And how do services such as family counseling impact these outcomes?

METHODS

Study Sample and Procedures

The study population consisted of adolescents, aged 13 to 19, recruited upon entering outpatient substance abuse treatment in Oregon and Washington State in 1998 and 1999. The original sampling protocol was designed to compare outcomes for publicly-funded treatment provided through managed care and through fee-for-service systems. Medicaid-eligible clients from 23 adolescent treatment agencies in demographically matched counties across Oregon and Washington participated. Participating treatment agencies provided group therapy, and most offered family therapy and individual therapy as needed; no uniformity of treatment protocol existed within or between agencies. Adolescent participants completed structured interviews at treatment admission and again at 6 months and 12 months past treatment admission.

Of the 328 adolescents recruited, 248 completed all 3 interviews (retention rate = 76%). Participants with complete data sets were included in the current analysis. Participants with complete data were more likely to be white and less likely to have been in school at the start of treatment than those with missing data. In stratifying the sample between those with a substance-abusing parent and those without, an additional 27 were excluded from the final analysis. These participants did not report a substance-abusing parent, but reported that another member of their household (typically a sibling or other peer) was an active substance abuser. Preliminary analyses suggested this cohort might differ from either of the other two groups. However, the cohort was too small in number to adequately investigate these differences and was therefore excluded from the analysis. The final sample consisted of 221 participants: 129 with a substance-abusing parent and 92 with no substance-abusing parent or other household member.

Measures

The study protocol featured several standardized instruments. The Youth Self Report Survey (YSR; Achenbach, 1991) measured mental health and social functioning. The YSR includes an internalizing problem scale measuring somatic, depressed, and anxious symptom sets, and an externalizing problem scale measuring aggressive and delinquent symptom sets. The Family Environment Scale (FES; Moos & Moos, 1994) measured family conflict and cohesion; treatment motivation was measured by a version of the Circumstances, Motivation, Readiness, and Suitability Scale (CMRS; DeLeon, Melnick, Kressel, & Jainchill, 1994) modified to exclude suitability variables. The adolescent version of the Addiction Severity Index (CASI-A; Meyers, McLellan, Jaeger, & Pettinati, 1995) measured substance use frequency; family, community, and personal stressors, and satisfaction with quality of life. The measure of substance use severity consisted of items based on the Diagnostic Statistical Manual of Mental Disorders IV (DSM-IV; American Psychiatric Association, 1994) and included items from the Substance Use Disorders Diagnostic Schedule IV (SUDDS-IV; Hoffman & Harrison, 1995). An algorithm developed by Dennis and Titus (2000) created a categorical variable consisting of no diagnosis, abuse, dependence, or physical dependence.

Protocol items also addressed demographics, selected risk factors for substance abuse, and treatment satisfaction. Treatment service use items asked whether participants received group therapy, individual therapy, and/or family therapy. Physical health status was measured using an index of general health complaints adapted from the SF-12 (Ware, Kosinski, & Keller, 1996). Peer drug use was indicated by the number of friends (up to 4) who had used or sold drugs in the previous 6 months.

Protocol items asking whether participants have a parent with a current or active alcohol or drug problem determined the study groups. Items did not specify whether the substance-abusing parent was male or female. For the purposes of this analysis, parents having an active alcohol or drug problem will be identified as *substance-abusing parents.*

Analysis

Participants were divided into 2 study groups: those with a substance-abusing parent and those with no substance-abusing parent or other household member. Differences between the study groups were assessed at baseline, 6 months, and at 12 months. Analyses were conducted to probe differences between the groups at each point in time, and within each group across the three time periods. Three tests were used to analyze differences between study groups, depending upon the scale of measurement of the dependent variable. For categorical outcomes (e.g., race), chi-square analyses were conducted. For ordinal outcomes (e.g., levels of use of alcohol and other drugs), Mann-Whitney U was employed. For continuous interval-level measures (e.g., externalizing psychosocial problems), analysis of variance (ANOVA) was used.

Within group differences for each study group were assessed from baseline to 6 months, 6 months to 12 months, and from baseline to 12 months. For ordinal dependent variables, the Friedman test was utilized with the Wilcoxon test for follow-up comparisons. For interval-level dependent variables repeated measures general linear modeling (GLM) was used along with paired sample t-test for follow-up comparisons. All analyses were conducted using the Statistical Package for the Social Sciences, Version 11.5 (SPSS, 11.5).

Logistic and linear regression were used to examine the relative contribution of family and individual counseling on 6-month and 12-month alcohol and marijuana outcomes and changes on Youth Self Report internalizing and externalizing scales. Independent variables entered in the model were study group, access to family counseling, and access to individual counseling. In the logistic regression analyses the two counseling variables were also included as separate interaction terms combined with study group.

RESULTS

Baseline Characteristics

Demographics and Background

A comparison between the two study groups at treatment entry revealed a number of differences in demographics and background variables (see Table 1). While the adolescent sample without a substance-abusing parent was disproportionately male, study participants with a substance-abusing parent were equally divided among males and females. Participants with a substance-abusing parent were more likely to be white than those without a substance-abusing parent. No significant differences existed between groups in age at the start of the treatment episode.

TABLE 1. Study Sample Characteristics

Baseline Characteristic	Substance Abusing Parent ($n = 129$)		No Substance Abusing Parent ($n = 92$)		*p*
	No.	%	No.	%	
Sex					$< .01^a$
Female	65	50%	28	30%	
Male	64	50%	64	70%	
Race/Ethnicity					$< .05^b$
White/Caucasian	95	74%	56	61%	
Racial minority[c]	34	26%	36	39%	
Mean Age	16		16		NS
Residence at treatment entry					NS
Controlled setting/Group home	19	15%	13	14%	
Family	79	61%	66	73%	
Foster parent	21	16%	9	10%	
Other	10	8%	4	3%	
Mean number of places lived in past 6 months	2.3		1.9		$< .01^d$
Arrested in lifetime	102	79%	66	72%	NS
Arrested in past 6 months	65	51%	40	43%	NS
On probation at treatment entry	67	52%	41	45%	NS
In school at start of treatment	109	84%	80	87%	NS
Mean physical heath problem score[e]	3.3		2.8		$< .01$

Note. NS = Not significant.
[a]$\chi^2(1) = 8.772$, $p < .01$. [b]$\chi^2(1) = 4.049$, $p < .05$. [c]Minority includes Asian, Black, Black Hispanic, Hispanic, American Indian, Other, multiracial, and respondents who provided more than one answer for ethnicity.
[d]$F(1,219) = 6.231$, $p < .01$. [e]Scale of 1 to 8. Higher number indicates greater number of health complaints.

At the time of treatment admission, no significant differences existed between the groups in place of residence. The majority of both samples lived with family members, with a sizeable minority living in alternative settings at treatment entry. However, study participants with a substance-abusing parent had greater housing instability in the six months prior to treatment in that they had lived in more settings. No significant differences appeared between the two study groups in criminal justice system involvement (arrests and probation). Additionally, no significant differences were found in the percent of participants attending school. Physical health status, however, differed significantly between groups with those with a substance-abusing parent reported a significantly higher number of health complaints in the previous 6 months.

Substance Use Indicators

A number of differences emerged between study groups in the area of substance use history (see Table 2). Participants with substance-abusing parents were significantly more likely to have a prior sub-

TABLE 2. Substance Use Indicators at Treatment Entry

Baseline Characteristics	Substance Abusing Parent (n = 129)		No Substance Abusing Parent (n = 92)		
	No.	%	No.	%	p
Prior treatment					
Inpatient/Residential	58	45%	24	26%	< .01[a]
Outpatient	107	83%	63	68%	< .01[b]
Substance use severity					NS
No diagnosis	24	19%	15	16%	
Abuse	30	23%	35	38%	
Dependence	7	5%	8	9%	
Physical dependence	68	53%	34	37%	
	M	*SD*	*M*	*SD*	
Age at first use					
Alcohol	10.69	3.58	11.77	2.43	< .01[c]
Marijuana	12.07	2.49	12.04	2.11	NS
Other drugs	13.97	1.42	13.84	1.58	NS
Readiness for treatment[d]	3.28	.60	3.18	.62	NS
Peer drug use[e]	1.78	1.14	1.50	1.11	NS

Note. NS = Not significant.
[a]$\chi^2(1) = 8.198$, $p < .01$. [b]$\chi^2(1) = 6.332$, $p < .01$. [c]$F(1,217) = 6.248$, $p < .01$. [d]Scale of 1 to 5, with 5 indicating greatest readiness for treatment. [e]Number of substance-using friends.

stance abuse inpatient or residential treatment episode and prior outpatient treatment history. While, substance use diagnostic severity at the start of the current treatment episode did not differ significantly between groups, an item-by-item analysis of diagnostic symptoms revealed significant differences in 7 of the 20 items, including physical withdrawal and binge substance use symptoms. In each case, participants with substance-abusing parents were more likely to report experiencing symptoms. These adolescents also had a significantly higher frequency of alcohol use and use of other drugs excluding marijuana in the 6 months prior to treatment admission (substance use frequency data appears in Tables 4 and 5). Marijuana was the most frequently used substance across study groups and no significant differences in marijuana use eixsted between groups. Adolescents with a substance-abusing parent were significantly younger at first use of alcohol, but not other drugs.

At the time of the current treatment admission, no significant differences existed between study groups in the area of treatment readiness and motivation. Additionally, no significant differences in peer drug use emerged between study groups.

Psychosocial and Stressor Indicators

The most pervasive differences between study groups appeared in the examination of psychosocial functioning, life stressors, and family dynamics (see Table 3). In general, adolescents with substance-abusing parents fared worse than those without substance-abusing parents. These adolescents were significantly more likely to have experienced family stressors and personal stressors in their lifetime, but not community stressors. Adolescents with substance-abusing parents reported significantly higher family conflict and lower family cohesion. Not surprisingly, adolescents in this group expressed significantly lower quality of life satisfaction.

In the area of psychosocial functioning (externalizing and internalizing problems measured by the Youth Self Report), participants with substance-abusing parents also exhibited significantly greater problems than their peers. Standardized YSR scores differed significantly overall and in internalizing and externalizing problems examined separately. A significantly greater percentage of adolescents with substance-abusing parents scored in the clinical range for both internalizing problems and externalizing problems.

TABLE 3. Psychosocial and Stressor Indicators at Treatment Entry

Baseline Characteristics	Substance Abusing Parent (n = 129)		No Substance Abusing Parent (n = 92)		p
	M	SD	M	SD	
Lifetime stressors					
Family	.67	.31	.56	.36	< .05[a]
Personal	.53	.22	.41	.22	< .01[b]
Community	.59	.34	.53	.37	NS
Family environment					
Family conflict	.53	.29	.35	.24	< .01[c]
Family Cohesion	.59	.30	.70	.25	< .01[d]
Life satisfaction	2.57	.63	2.80	.60	< .01[e]
	No.	%	No.	%	
Internalizing problems					< .01[f]
Normal/Average	91	71%	81	88%	
Borderline	13	10%	6	7%	
Clinical	25	19%	5	5%	
Externalizing problems					< .01[g]
Normal/Average	45	35%	48	52%	
Borderline	23	18%	19	21%	
Clinical	61	47%	25	27%	

Note. NS = Not significant.
[a]$F(1,219) = 5.605$, $p < .05$. [b]$F(1,219) = 15.546$, $p < .01$. [c]$F(1,218) = 24.281$, $p < .01$. [d]$F(1,218) = 9.389$, $p < .01$. [e]$F(1,219) = 7.015$, $p < .01$. [f]$\chi^2 (2, n = 221) = 10.596$, $p < .01$. [g]$\chi^2 (2, n = 221) = 9.623$, $p < .01$.

Treatment Variables

At the 6 month interview, participants were asked about their experiences in the treatment episode through which they joined the study. The questions focused on participation in family and individual counseling and treatment satisfaction.

Family and Individual Counseling

Participants with a substance-abusing parent were significantly more likely to have participated in counseling or therapy with another family member during treatment than those without a substance-abusing parent [30% v 17%; $\chi^2(2 = 4.801$, $p < .05$]. Adolescents with a substance-abusing parent were also significantly more likely to receive individual counseling sessions [77% v 62%; $\chi^2(1) = 6.076$, $p < .01$], though the majority of both study groups reported having received individual sessions. Almost all (95%) of the study participants received group therapy.

Treatment Satisfaction

There were no significant differences between study groups in treatment satisfaction. Both groups were equally highly satisfied with access to treatment and the helpfulness of the services in dealing with substance use, emotional problems, and other life issues. No differences appeared in either the overall treatment satisfaction, or in any of the 12 individual satisfaction items.

Outcomes

Substance Use Outcomes

Though outcomes were similar for alcohol and for other drugs excluding marijuana, prevalence of other drug use was quite low. For this reason, we have limited our discussion here to alcohol and marijuana use. Though participants with substance-abusing parents evidenced significantly greater frequency of alcohol use ($p < .01$) at treatment entry, both study groups showed declines in their substance use over time. Both groups demonstrated significant improvement in substance abuse from baseline to 6 months at the $p < .01$ level for both alcohol and marijuana. Although no further improvement was seen from 6 months to 12 months the initial improvement was maintained at 12 months for both groups. Participants with a substance-abusing parent evidenced a greater degree of change than participants without a substance-abusing parent. A separate analysis revealed that significant baseline differences between study groups in frequency of alcohol use disappeared at the 6 and 12 month data points. Marijuana use did not differ significantly between study groups at any data point. Tables 4 and 5 illustrate alcohol and marijuana use outcomes over the course of the study.

Logistic regression analyses were conducted to examine the relationship between individual and family counseling and substance use outcomes. Analysis of 6 month outcomes revealed important differences between the two study groups in the effect of the counseling on alcohol use, but not marijuana use. For both study groups, family and individual counseling appeared to have no impact on alcohol or marijuana use at 12 months past treatment entry.

In alcohol use outcomes at the 6 month interview, adolescents with a substance-abusing parent were nearly 3 times more likely to achieve a positive outcome (i.e., consume less or remain abstinent) than adoles-

TABLE 4. Alcohol Use Outcomes

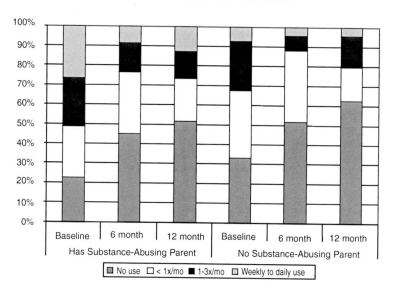

Note: HSAP = Has Substance-Abusing Parent, NSAP = No Substance-Abusing Parent
<u>Between group alcohol use comparisons by data point</u>
Baseline: z = −2.344, p < .05 (HSAP > NSAP)
6-mo: z = −1.241, NS (HSAP = NSAP)
12-mo: z = −1.548, NS (HSAP = NSAP)
<u>Within group change over time</u>
HSAP   Baseline to 6-mo.: z = −5.403, p < .01 (↓ use)
      6-mo to 12-mo: z = −7.39, NS (= use)
NSAP   Baseline to 6-mo: z = −4.303, p < .01 (↓ use)
      6-mo to 12-mo: z = −.033, NS (= use)

cents without a substance-abusing parent. This effect is likely to be due to the fact that a greater percentage of adolescents with substance-abusing parents enter treatment with more severe alcohol problems. Of greater relevance, however, is the influence of family counseling on 6 month alcohol use for adolescents with substance-abusing parents. Specifically, adolescents with a substance-abusing parent who received family counseling were half as likely to achieve a positive outcome at 6 months than adolescents with a substance-abusing parent who did not receive family counseling. In contrast, adolescents without a substance-abusing parent who received family counseling were nearly 3 times more likely to have a positive outcome compared to adolescents without a substance abusing parent who did not receive family counseling.

TABLE 5. Marijuana Use Outcomes

| | No use | □ < 1x/mo | ■ 1-3 x/mo | □ Weekly to daily use |

Note: HSAP = Has Substance-Abusing Parent, NSAP = No Substance-Abusing Parent Between group marijuana use comparisons by data point
Baseline: $z = -.112$, NS (HSAP = NSAP)
6-mo: $z = -.502$, NS (HSAP = NSAP)
12-mo: $z = -.551$, NS (HSAP = NSAP)
Within group change over time
HSAP   Baseline to 6-mo: $z = -5.612$, $p < .01$ (↓ use)
     6-mo to 12-mo: $z = -2.061$, NS (= use)
NSAP   Baseline to 6-mo: $z = -4.8$, $p < .01$ (↓ use)
     6-mo to 12-mo: $z = -3.52$, NS (= use)

Unlike alcohol outcomes, 6 month marijuana outcomes were more affected by individual counseling than by family counseling, and parental substance abuse appeared to be inconsequential. In general, adolescents in both study groups who received individual counseling were greater than 2.5 times more likely to achieve positive outcomes at 6 months than adolescents who did not receive individual counseling.

Psychosocial Outcomes

For psychosocial functioning outcomes, both externalizing and internalizing problem scores were examined. For externalizing problems, both groups showed significant improvement (reduced problems) at the 6 month interview and this improvement was maintained at the 12 month interview. Nevertheless, externalizing problems were the only outcome area measured in which participants with substance-abusing parents maintained significantly greater severity compared to those without substance-abusing parents at both 6 and 12 month interviews. Table 6 displays the percent of adolescents scoring in the clinical problem range for both externalizing and internalizing problems at each data point.

Both study groups reported lower rates of internalizing problems than externalizing ones. Little change occurred over time in internaliz-

TABLE 6. Psychosocial Outcomes

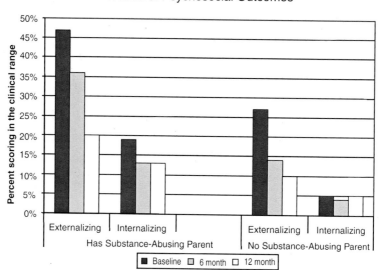

Note: HSAP = Has Substance-Abusing Parent, NSAP = No Substance-Abusing Parent
Between group externalizing problems by data point
Baseline: $z = -3.034$, $p < .01$ (HSAP > NSAP)
6-mo: $z = -3.343$, $p < .01$ (HSAP > NSAP)
12-mo: $z = -3.07$, $p < .01$ (HSAP > NSAP)
Within group externalizing change over time
HSAP   Baseline to 6-mo: $z = -3.479$, $p < .01$ ($\downarrow$ pblms)
       6-mo to 12-mo: $z = -2.272$, NS (= pblms)
NSAP   Baseline to 6-mo: $z = -3.734$, $p < .01$ ($\downarrow$ pblms)
       6-mo to 12-mo: $z = -.638$, NS (= pblms)
Between group internalizing problems by data point
Baseline: $z = -3.183$, $p < .01$ (HSAP > NSAP)
6-mo: $z = -3.300$, $p < .01$ (HSAP > NSAP)
12-mo: $z = -1.931$, NS (HSAP = NSAP)
Within group internalizing change over time
HSAP   Baseline to 6-mo: $z = -2.490$, NS (= pblms)
       6-mo to 12-mo: $z = -.632$, NS (= pblms)
NSAP   Baseline to 6-mo: $z = -1.466$, NS (= pblms)
       6-mo to 12-mo: $z = -3.52$, NS (= use)

ing problems for either group; improvement was not significant in either case, although participants with substance-abusing parents did improve (reduce problems) slightly. Adolescents with substance-abusing parents reported greater internalizing problems than their peers at baseline and at 6 months, but differences were not significant at the 12 month interview.

Linear regression analyses suggested that internalizing and externalizing problems were differentially affected by parental substance abuse, type of counseling received, and time. Adolescents with substance-abusing parents were significantly more likely to have higher internalizing problem scores at the 6 month interview and higher externalizing problem scores at both 6 and 12 month interviews than adolescents without substance-abusing parents even after baseline scores were statistically controlled. Interestingly, only 12 month internalizing scores appeared to be influenced by type of counseling received and this effect was limited to adolescents with substance-abusing parents. Specifically, adolescents with substance-abusing parents were significantly more likely to show improvements in internalization problems if they received individual counseling whereas the internalization problems of adolescents without substance-abusing parents were not affected by individual counseling.

DISCUSSION

This study found that adolescents with substance-abusing parents enter treatment with greater problem severity than their peers in a number of areas, including greater housing instability, poorer physical health status, greater lifetime stressor ratings, poorer family functioning scores, lower quality of life satisfaction, and lower psychosocial functioning. Adolescents with substance-abusing parents exhibited no significant differences from their peers in criminal justice involvement, peer drug use, school attendance, or treatment readiness.

Substance-related measures at treatment admission presented a mixed picture, though the differences were in the direction of greater problems among adolescents with substance-abusing parents. Such adolescents presented with a greater likelihood of prior treatment history, younger age at first use of alcohol (but not other drugs), and greater likelihood of having experienced many substance use consequences (though no differences in overall diagnostic severity). Interestingly, adolescents with substance-abusing parents reported greater frequency of alcohol use and other drug use, but no differences in frequency of marijuana use.

National surveys have identified an upward trend in adolescent marijuana use in the last decade (Dennis, Babor, Roebuck, & Donaldson, 2002; Substance Abuse and Mental Health Services Administration, 2003), and this general trend appears to supercede the mediating influence of parental substance abuse for this clinical sample. It is possible that the prevalence of peer marijuana use and decreases in perceived harmfulness and disapproval (Johnston, O'Malley, Bachman, & Schulenberg, 2003) may override parental influence.

Substance use outcomes were positive for both groups, and those with substance-abusing parents closed the gap between themselves and other adolescents in alcohol and non-marijuana drug use. Importantly, both groups were able to maintain substance use improvements at the 12 month follow-up, when almost all were no longer receiving treatment. The similarity between the study groups in motivation at treatment entry and satisfaction with the treatment received may be relevant, as the literature links both factors to treatment retention and outcomes for adolescents (Cady, Winters, Jordan, Solberg, & Stinchfield, 1996; Druss, Rosenheck, & Stolar, 1999; McLellan & Hunkeler, 1998).

Perhaps the most unanticipated finding was the impact of family counseling on alcohol use outcomes. For adolescents with no substance-abusing parent, family counseling had a positive short-term effect (abstinence or decreased alcohol use). However, for adolescents with a substance-abusing parent, family counseling had a negative short-term effect (increased or maintained alcohol use). This intriguing result requires further study. It is possible that parent engagement interventions other than family counseling are indicated for adolescents with substance-abusing parents. It may be that because alcohol use is socially condoned, substance-abusing parents minimize its negative consequences. Also of interest is the finding that marijuana use patterns were unrelated to either parental substance abuse or family counseling, although individual counseling did appear to improve outcomes. This suggests that the social and contextual functions of adolescent marijuana use may differ from those of alcohol or other drugs. Research currently emerging from the Cannabis Youth Treatment Trials will continue to expand the knowledge base, examining treatment effectiveness, individual subtypes, and other aspects specific to adolescent marijuana users (Babor, Webb, Burleson, & Kaminer, 2002; Dennis, 2004).

Externalizing problems also improved for both groups, though work appears needed in closing the gap between groups. The strong link in the literature between adolescent substance use disorders and external-ing problems, and the relationship between parental substance abuse and externalizing problems, suggest this as an important area for further research. Internalizing problems, though less prevalent in the sample studied here, proved more intransigent and may require different, perhaps more mental health-focused interventions.

STUDY LIMITATIONS

Limitations to these analyses exist. We are unable to isolate parental substance use as the key contributing factor in study group differences at treatment entry. As data about parental mental health status (including antisocial personality disorder) were not collected, it cannot be determined if parental co-occurring disorders played a role in study group differences. Baseline differences in gender and race between study groups were found. Those with a substance-abusing parent were more likely to be Caucasian and female than those without a substance-abusing parent. The literature has not generally shown evidence of differences in substance use outcomes due to gender or race (Brower & Carey, 2003; Foster, Peters, & Marshall, 2000), although treatment needs often differ. While the largest percentage of study participants were aged 15 to 16, study samples included adolescent treatment clients from age 13 to 19. Differences in treatment response based on age may exist, but were beyond the scope of this study. Another limitation in assessing treatment outcomes is the lack of data regarding intensity and duration of treatment services. In particular, lack of data regarding the family therapy utilized by participating agencies (including dosage, philosophy, and protocol) limits interpretation. While differences in treatment effectiveness may exist between agencies, the two study groups were represented in approximately equal proportions within agencies. In general, participating agencies used eclectic rather than manual-guided family therapy models. Whether results related to family therapy would differ based on the use of specific protocols cannot be determined here.

CONCLUSION

This study indicates that current adolescent treatment practice is effective in stimulating sustainable changes in substance use and emotional/behavioral health for adolescents with substance-abusing parents. This general indication of treatment effectiveness and provision of family services suggest that adolescent treatment approaches are evolving to the specific concerns of adolescents, rather than simply replicating adult treatment models. As a system-wide investigation in two states, the current study did not attempt to examine the therapeutic models in use at the participating treatment agencies. Further research is needed to isolate the elements responsible for effecting change and the mechanisms by which the change occurs. In particular, research is needed to determine the effects of family-level interventions on outcomes for adolescents with substance-abusing parents.

There is some evidence that treatment providers are cognizant of the particular challenges of working with this population. While it is certain that many counselors and social workers are addressing parental substance abuse in their work with adolescents, it is unlikely that consistency in approach has been attained given the gap in knowledge in this area. It is clear that theory development and interventions will continue to evolve, and evidence-based technologies will expand for addressing the treatment needs of adolescents with substance-abusing parents. If our sample is representative of adolescent treatment populations, attention to this issue is critical: fully half the adolescents in our sample were children of active substance abusers. For social workers and counselors, it may be useful to know that, while adolescents whose parents are active substance abusers fuse treatment as their peers.

REFERENCES

Achenbach, T.M. (1991). *Manual for the Child Behavior Checklist 4-18, 1991 Profile.* Burlington: University of Vermont, Department of Psychiatry.

American Psychiatric Association. (1994). *Diagnostic and statistical manual of mental disorders* (4th ed.). Washington, DC: Author.

Anda, R.F., Whitfield, C.L., Felitti, V.J., Chapman, D., Edwards, V.J., Dube, S.R. et al. (2002). Adverse childhood experiences, alcoholic parents, and later risk alcoholism and depression. *Journal of Psychiatric Services, 53*(8), 1001-1009.

Babor, T.F., Webb, C., Burleson, J.A., & Kaminer, Y. (2002). Subtypes for classifying adolescents with marijuana use disorders: Construct validity and clinical implications. *Addiction, 97*(Suppl 1), 58-69.

Brower, K.J., & Care, T.L., (2003). Racially related health disparities and alcoholism treatment outcomes. *Alcoholism: Clinical and Experimental Research, 27*(8), 1365-1367.

Cady, M.E., Winters, K.C., Jordan, D.A., Solberg, K.B., & Stinchfield, R.D. (1996). Motivation to change as a predictor of treatment outcome for adolescent substance abusers. *Journal of Child & Adolescent Substance Abuse, 5*, 73-91.

Catalano, R.F., Gainey, R.R., Fleming, C.B., Haggerty, K.P., & Johnson, N.O. (1999). An experimental intervention with families of substance abuser one-year follow-up of the focus on families project. *Addiction, 94*(2), 241-4.

Chassin, L., Pitts, S.C., DeLucia, C., & Todd, M. (1999). A longitudinal study of children of alcoholics: Predicting young adult substance use disorders, anxiety, and depression. *Journal of Abnormal Psychology, 108*(1), 106-119.

Coatsworth, J.D., Santisteban, D.A., McBride, C.K., & Szapocznik, J. (2001). Brief strategic family therapy versus community control: Engagement, retention, and an exploration of the moderating role of adolescent symptom severity. *Family Process, 40*, 313-332.

DeLeon, G., Melnick, G., Kressel, D., & Jainchill, N. (1994). Circumstances, motivation, readiness, and suitability (The CMRS Scales): Predicting retention in therapeutic community treatment. *American Journal of Drug and Alcohol Abuse, 20*(4), 495-515.

Dennis M.L., & Titus, J. (2000). *Patterns of adolescent substance dependence, abuse, and use.* Paper presented at The 108th Annual Convention of the American Psychological Association; Washington, DC.

Dennis, M., Babor, T.F., Roebuck, M.C., & Donaldson, J. (2002). Changing the focus: the case for recognizing and treating cannabis use disorders. *Addiction, 97*(1), 4-15.

Dennis, M.L. (2004, April). *Developing effective drug treatment for adolescents: Results from the Cannabis Youth Treatment (CYT) trials.* Poster session presented at the American Society of Addiction Medicine 2004 Annual Conference, Washington, DC.

Druss, B.G., Rosenheck, R.A., & Stolar, M. (1999). Patient satisfaction and administrative measures as indicators of the quality of mental health care. *Psychiatric Services, 50*(8), 1053-1058.

Edwards, M., & Steinglass, P. (1995). Family therapy treatment outcomes for alcoholism. *Journal of Marital & Family Therapy, 21*(4), 475-509.

Ellis, D.A., Zucker, R.A., & Fitzgerald, H.E. (1997). The role of family influences in development and risk. *Alcohol Health & Research World, 21*(3), 218-226.

Foster, J.H., Peters, T.J., & Marshall, E.J. (2000). Quality of life measures and outcome in alcohol-dependent men and women. *Alcohol, 22*(1), 45-52.

Friedman, A., & Utada, A. (1992). The family environments of adolescent drug abusers. *Family Dynamics of Addiction Quarterly, 2*(2), 32-45.

Godley, S.H., Meyers, R.J., Smith, J.E., Karvinen, T., Titus, J.C., Godley, M.D. et al. (2001). *Cannabis youth treatment (CYT) series, Vol. 4. The adolescent community reinforcement approach for adolescent cannabis users* (DHHS Publication No. 01-3489). Rockville, MD: Center for Substance Abuse Treatment.

Hoffman, N.G., & Harrison, P.A. (1995). *Substance use disorders diagnostic schedule* (4th ed.). St. Paul, MN: New Standards.

Johnson, J.L., & Leff, M. (1999). Children of substance abusers: Overview of research findings. *Pediatrics, 103*(5), 1085-1099.

Johnston, L.D., O'Malley, P.M., Bachman, J.G., & Schulenberg, J.E. (2003). *Monitoring the Future national survey results on drug use, 1975-2003: Volume I: Secondary school students* (NIH Publication No. 04-5507). Bethesda, MD: National Institute on Drug Abuse.

Liddle, H.A., Dakof, G.A., Parker, K., Diamond, G.S., Barrett, K., & Tejeda, M. (2001). Multidimensional Family Therapy for adolescent drug abuse: Results of a randomized clinical trial. *American Journal of Drug and Alcohol Abuse, 27*, 651-688.

McLellan, A.T., & Hunkeler, E: (1998). Patient satisfaction and outcomes in alcohol and drug abuse treatment. *Psychiatric Services, 49*(5), 573-575.

Menees, M.M., & Segrin, C. (2000). The specificity of disrupted processes in families of adult children of alcoholics. *Alcohol* (4), 361-367.

Meyers, K., McLellan, A.T., Jaeger, J.L., & Pettinati, H.M. (1995). The development of the Comprehensive Addiction Severity Index for Adolescents (CASI-A): An interview for assessing multiple problems of adolescents. *Journal of Substance Abuse Treatment, 12*(3), 181-193.

Moos, R.H., & Moos, B.S. (1994). *Family Environment Scale manual: Development applications, research* (3rd ed.). Palo Alto, CA: Consulting Psychologists Press.

Ozechowski, T.J., & Liddle, H.A. (2000). Family-based therapy for adolescent drug abuse: Knowns and unknowns. *Clinical Child and Family Psychology Review, 3*(4), 269-298.

Puttler, L.I., Zucker, R.Z., Fitzgerald, H.E., & Bingham, C.R. (1998). Behavioral outcomes among children of alcoholics during the early and middle childhood years: Familial subtype variations. *Alcohol: Clinical and Experimental Research, 22*(9), 1962- 1972.

Rowe, C.L., & Liddle, H.A. (2003). Substance abuse. *Journal of Marital Family Therapy, 29*(1), 97-120.

Schuckit, M.A., Smith, T.L., Radziminski, S., & Heyneman, E.K. (2000). Behavioral symptoms and psychiatric diagnoses among 162 children in nonalcoholic or alcoholic families. *American Journal of Psychiatry, 157*(11), 1881-1883.

Sher, K.J. (1991). Psychological characteristics of children of alcoholics: Overview of research methods and findings. In M. Galanter (Ed.), *Recent developments in alcoholism: Volume 9. Children of alcoholics* (pp. 301-321). New York: Plenum Press.

Sher, K.J. (1997). Psychological characteristics of children of alcoholics. *Alcohol Health & Research World, 21*(3), 247-4.

Stanger, C., Kamon, J., Dumenci, L., Higgins, S.T., Bickel, W.K., Grabowski, J. et al. (2002). Predictors of internalizing and externalizing problems among children of cocaine and opiate dependent parents. *Drug and Alcohol Dependence, 66*(2), 199-212.

Substance Abuse and Mental Health Services Administration, Office of Applied Studies. (2003). *Results from the 2002 National Survey on Drug Use and Health: National findings* (DHHS Publication No. SMA 03-3836). Rockville, MD: Author.

Ware, J.E., Kosinski, M., & Keller, S.D. (1996). A 12-Item Short-Form Health Survey: Construction of scales and preliminary tests of reliability and validity. *Medical Care, 34*(3), 220-233.

Zucker, R. (1994). Pathways to alcohol problems and alcoholism: A developmental account of the evidence for multiple alcoholisms and for contextual contributions to risk. In R. Zucker, G. Boyd, & J. Howard (Eds.), *The development of alcohol problems: Exploring the biopsychosocial matrix of risk* (pp. 5-290; NIAAA Research Monograph No. 26). Rockville, MD: National Institutes of Health.

SPECIAL TOPICS:
REFLECTIONS FROM THE FIELD

Student Assistance Programs:
An Interview with Ellen Morehouse

This interview was conducted by Lori K. Holleran

Morehouse: The Westchester **Student Assistance Program (SAP)** began in 1979 as an adaptation of the Employee Assistance Program (EAP) model for secondary schools. EAPs have been used successfully by industry to assist employees whose work performance has been negatively affected by alcohol, other drugs, or personal and family problems. The Westchester SAP model places experienced, specially trained counselors in each school to implement universal, selective, and indicated program

Ellen Morehouse, LCSW, CASAC, CPP, is Executive Director, Student Assistance Services, Tarrytown, NY. She is the creator of three national model alcohol and drug abuse prevention and early intervention programs and has been the recipient of grants from the NIAAA, CDC, CSAP, OJJDP, and U.S. Department of Education. Lori K. Holleran, MSW, ACSW, PhD, is Assistant Professor, School of Social Work, University of Texas, Austin. She is Special Topics Editor for the Journal.

[Haworth co-indexing entry note]: "Student Assistance Programs: An Interview with Ellen Morehouse." Holleran, Lori K. Co-published simultaneously in *Journal of Social Work Practice in the Addictions* (The Haworth Press, Inc.) Vol. 6, No. 1/2, 2006, pp. 175-180; and: *Impact of Substance Abuse on Children and Families: Research and Practice Implications* (ed: Shulamith Lala Ashenberg Straussner, and Christine Huff Fewell) The Haworth Press, Inc., 2006, pp. 175-180. Single or multiple copies of this article are available for a fee from The Haworth Document Delivery Service [1-800-HAWORTH, 9:00 a.m. - 5:00 p.m. (EST). E-mail address: docdelivery@ haworthpress.com].

doi:10.1300/J160v06n01_09

components. This means that student assistance counselors provide: school-wide awareness (universal) activities; services to students at higher risk for substance abuse, such as students with alcoholic and drug abusing parents or siblings (selective); and services for students who are already using substances (indicated). Activities include: information dissemination; normative education; resistance skills; social competency skills; communications skills; coping, stress and anger management; problem-solving/decision-making; and problem identification and referral. These activities are conducted by the Student Assistance Counselor, primarily in small group and individual sessions. Student Assistance Counselors also work with students, school administrators, parents, and community groups on environmental approaches to change attitudes and behaviors. The Westchester SAP has been effective in assisting adolescents by both preventing and reducing alcohol and drug-related problems. It was designated as a program for replication by the National Institute on Alcoholism and Alcohol Abuse in 1982 and has been replicated in schools throughout the United States. Nationally, there are three models of SAP. The Westchester model uses professionals employed by a community based non-profit or public agency with expertise in substance abuse prevention and early intervention. The counselor is supervised jointly by the school principal and by a clinical or program supervisor at the agency. The second model uses a professional employed by the school and either supervised by an outside agency and school employee or not supervised by an outside agency. The third model called the core team model uses existing school staff that receives some training, but has student assistance team duties in addition to teaching, counseling, or administrative responsibilities. The core team model results in fewer self referrals, sees fewer students, and is much less expensive because existing school staff is being used instead of hiring a new full or part time master's level professional. SAPs are being implemented in at least some schools in all 50 states.

In 1988, a five-year high-risk youth grant from the Center for Substance Abuse Prevention funded the implementation and adaptation of the SAP in residential childcare facilities. The Residential Student Assistance Program (RSAP) was designed for adolescents placed in residential childcare facilities because they have committed violent or delinquent acts, have been physically, sexually, or psychologically abused, have experienced chronic failure in school, and/or have experienced mental health problems including attempted suicide. These adolescents have multiple risk factors for substance use including a history of early substance use and have a parent that abuses substances. Most of the residents fall somewhere on the continuum from experimentation to dependency. These adolescents tend to "fall between the cracks" of the substance abuse prevention system for youth. Because of their difficulties, they generally do not attend school regularly and miss exposure to the in-school substance abuse prevention curricula. The nature of their problems results in their inability to remain at home or in a foster home and requires high levels of state mandated services of which substance abuse prevention services are often at the end of a long list of priorities. Furthermore, at typical residential facilities, there are limited, if any, direct substance abuse prevention, education, and early intervention services available. The RSAP represents a combination of interventions designed to address the unique needs of this underserved population while they are a "captive audience."

Project SUCCESS (**S**chools **U**tilizing **C**oordinated **C**ommunity **E**fforts to **S**trengthen **S**tudents) is an adaptation of the RSAP, for alternative schools. It was first implemented as a result of a three-year CSAP grant in 1996. Students are enrolled in alternative schools for problems related to poor academic performance, truancy, discipline problems, and negative attitudes toward school, which places them at high risk for substance abuse in adolescence.

Project SUCCESS is unique in that it targets youths who have more risk factors than adolescents attending regular schools but who are not as high risk as the adolescents that have been removed from "family" (when there was a family), school, and community. The adolescents targeted for Project SUCCESS are in the middle of the adolescent risk continuum. For most, Alternative school is their last chance for a non-institutionalized education. Many could end up, or have already been, in the juvenile justice, correction, psychiatric, or foster care systems; all are living in the community and are not institutionalized; and the great majority is living with at least one biological, adoptive, or foster parent. This means that these youth have access to services in the community; they have freedom of movement; and there is access to a "parent." Project SUCCESS is currently being replicated in schools in 18 states.

All three programs are science-based programs that build on the findings of other successful prevention programs by using interventions that are effective in reducing risk factors and enhancing protective factors. The targeted risk and protective factors were identified through a series of separate focus groups conducted with students, parents of students, and school and residential staff. In addition, a review of the literature was conducted to determine the state-of-the-art in substance abuse prevention strategies.

The programs are based on the well-documented prevention principles that delaying the onset of substance use and reducing use in youth can be accomplished by:

- Increasing perception of risk of harm.
- Changing adolescents' norms and expectations about substance use.
- Building and enhancing social and resistance skills.
- Changing community norms and values regarding substance use.
- Fostering and enhancing resiliency and protective factors, especially in high risk youth.

In addition, the following conclusions are central to the program's philosophy:

- Students who are introduced to the pressures they will encounter to use substances and taught the skills to resist these pressures are less likely to use substances (Evans et al., 1981).
- Intervention programs must be tailored to the developmental stage of the adolescent participants. Substance use can be seen as a way to lessen the pain associated with different developmental tasks (Kandel, 1980), and psychological or social states (Kumpfer and Turner, 1991).
- Correcting erroneous normative beliefs about substance use and modeling conservative norms are important ingredients of prevention and early intervention programs (Hansen and Graham, 1998).
- While involving parents in school-based programs can positively reinforce in school messages (Pentz et al., 1989) and help facilitate adolescent change (Bry, 1997), it has been shown that adolescents can have positive change without familial involvement (Tobler et al., 1992; NIAA, 1984; Kleinman et al., 1992, Klitzner et al., 1990) and that familial involvement may be counter productive (Glynn, 1989).
- Highly skilled leaders and involvement in group sessions are two of the most important factors in the effectiveness of prevention programs (Tobler, 1992).

RSAP used a quasi-experimental design to evaluate the program's effectiveness by comparing program participants with a comparison group. Adolescents in the treatment group showed dramatic reductions in the use of alcohol, tobacco, and marijuana from pre- to post-test measures, while in-house comparison youth showed relatively unchanged rates of use.

Project SUCCESS had a more rigorous evaluation and used random assignment to intervention conditions in addition to comparison sites. Project SUCCESS was highly effective in reducing ATOD use. There was a statistically significant 37% reduction in the rate of use by the Project SUCCESS program youth when compared to the non-program youth.

Both RSAP and Project SUCCESS have been designated as Exemplary Model Programs by the Substance Abuse and Mental Health Services Administration (SAMHSA) and, to my knowledge, are the only two model programs that target adolescents with substance abusing parents. More information can be obtained by going to the SAMHSA Model Program website (*www.samhsa.gov*).

Holleran: What is the value of your program and similar programs?

Morehouse: The value of the programs is that they prevent and reduce substance abuse in adolescents. They are one of the few easily accessible places where teens with substance abusing parents as well as teens who are using substances can go for help with these issues.

Holleran: What are the challenges and down-sides of such programs for children?

Morehouse: The challenges for teens are discussing emotionally laden issues for a class period and then having to go to math class. The only "down-side" is occasional insensitivity from teachers about missing a class, and the very small risk of breach of confidentiality by a friend or counseling group member.

Holleran: Who are the most indicated facilitators of such programs and why? What training do you recommend that they receive in order to implement with this population?

Morehouse: MSWs with group skills and skills in working with adolescents are the ideal candidates for these types of programs. Their training in psychosocial assessment combined with their understanding of family systems provides a context for understanding how COSAPs are impacted by their parents' behavior and informs their interventions with these teens.

Holleran: If a social worker or agency wants to start such a program, what recommendations would you make for them to be successful?

Morehouse: Make sure the principal of the school and the superintendent of the school district understand the program and believe in its importance. Have the principal interview the finalists for the position and select who will be her/his Student Assistance or Project SUCCESS counselor. When possible, it is helpful for an assistant principal and member of the pupil personnel team (guidance counselor, school social worker, or psychologist) to also be part of the interview and decision making process. Also, purchase the implementation manual for the program and attend the three-day training, if possible. The higher the degree of fidelity in program implementation, the more likely positive results will be achieved.

Holleran: What do you think the future directions for services to children of addicts/alcoholics need to be?

Morehouse: Prevention programs need to evaluate their impact on children of alcoholics/addicts. Too often a "one size fits all" approach is being used and we don't know if this population most at risk for substance abuse is benefiting from the program.

Holleran: Can our readers contact you if they want further information or direction? AND/OR, what resources should our readers utilized if they need more information or direction?

Morehouse: If readers want more information about Project SUCCESS or RSAP, they should first go to the *www.samhsa.gov* website and click on National Registry of Evidenced Based Programs and Practices (NREP), and then click on Model Programs. For more specific questions, they should call Student Assistance Services Corp. at (914) 332-1300, speak to the receptionist, and then she will direct the caller to one of our supervisors or to me. For information about training, readers can go to our website at *www.sascorp.org*.

ENDPAGE

Partners and Adult Children of Alcoholics in Online Treatment

Elizabeth Zelvin

Those who seek professional help online often cite relationship, marital, and family issues as the stated presenting problem. Many of them either grew up in an alcoholic family or have an intimate relationship with an alcohol or other substance abuser. The online therapist with training and experience in addictions has an effective key to open the door to significant work through text-based treatment.

Online clients may choose to work via e-mail or chat or a combination of the two. E-mail is a challenge for the therapist because it requires sustained narrative, very unlike the clinician's role in office practice. The online therapist must strike a balance, avoiding both unresponsive silence and overly directive advice. E-mail provides an opportunity to do many things at once: ask questions for assessment and exploration,

Elizabeth Zelvin, LCSW, ACSW, CASAC, C-CATODSW, is Online Clinician, *www.LZcybershrink.com*, and conducts training for therapists in online clinical skills.

[Haworth co-indexing entry note]: "Partners and Adult Children of Alcoholics in Online Treatment." Zelvin, Elizabeth. Co-published simultaneously in *Journal of Social Work Practice in the Addictions* (The Haworth Press, Inc.) Vol. 6, No. 1/2, 2006, pp. 181-185; and: *Impact of Substance Abuse on Children and Families: Research and Practice Implications* (ed: Shulamith Lala Ashenberg Straussner, and Christine Huff Fewell) The Haworth Press, Inc., 2006, pp. 181-185. Single or multiple copies of this article are available for a fee from The Haworth Document Delivery Service [1-800-HAWORTH, 9:00 a.m. - 5:00 p.m. (EST). E-mail address: docdelivery@haworthpress.com].

doi:10.1300/J160v06n01_10

interpret the client's material, provide psychoeducation about dysfunctional systems and models of recovery, and elicit and support feelings. Chat operates a lot more like office practice, although it takes place in text instead of spoken words. The therapeutic relationship that quickly springs to life can be used to provide a corrective experience to adult children of alcoholic and neglectful or abusive parents and model healthy relationships for the significant others of addicted or otherwise dysfunctional partners.

Some online clients, like their face-to-face counterparts, reach out only when they are in crisis. Because the Internet transcends geography, individuals who might otherwise have difficulty obtaining the help they need have access to information, resources, and support.

Sally, a farmer's wife, contacted me when her alcoholic husband resumed drinking only a few days after his return from detox. She lived on an isolated farm many miles from the nearest town. She had heard of Al-Anon but could not attend meetings, as the nearest was two hours' drive away. There were no therapists or treatment programs within a reasonable distance. Nor could her family provide support.

In desperation, Sally reached out on the Internet. Our e-mail exchanges provided her the opportunity to tell her story, express her feelings, reality test in a situation that became increasingly chaotic, and learn more about alcoholism and its effects on the family as well as solutions and resources. Just as I would have in office practice, I validated her feelings, helped her problem solve with respect to her life situation, and helped her develop ego strength and reinforce healthy boundaries. I also helped her find an online Al-Anon group for additional support. Sally was one of many who find they can use the therapist's e-mails as a transitional object or representation of the therapist in between sessions. She wrote: "I just reread your last message for about the tenth time. It helps me get back to where I need to be."

Gloria, in contrast to Sally, did not mention alcohol at all when she e-mailed me for help. She wrote that "ugly and destructive patterns of communication" between herself and her husband were being repeated between him and their teenaged son. She also reported that her younger son, a ten-year-old, played the role of mediator with what sounded to me like the excessive maturity of a parentified child. My addiction specialist's antennae went up. In exploring the possibilities for her husband's explosive, impulsive, and often childish behavior, I asked if he was drinking. I also addressed her own response to the situation, shifting the focus from her concern for the other family members to her own needs:

I suspect you feel angry, scared, sad, lonely, disappointed, and helpless. Are those on target? You need to take care of yourself, because if you're running on empty, you won't have the energy to do anything for those you love.

Gloria's reply included a long history of her husband's drinking, which she called "the elephant in the living room" without being aware that this phrase is frequently used for an alcoholic situation in which the family is in denial. By the time she wrote her third e-mail, she had attended her first Al-Anon meeting and was determined to help the whole family address the issue.

Adult children of alcoholics (ACOA) present with depression, grief and loss issues, and eating disorders, as well as relationship problems. A blend of psychoeducation, supportive therapy, and psychodynamic exploration, along with whatever connection can be made with appropriate 12-step programs online or in the client's community, goes a long way toward alleviating the client's pain and effecting change and growth.

Karen worked with me in weekly chat sessions. She was an ACOA whose father had been sober for many years. Although he no longer drank, he remained silent and emotionally distant, expressing affection only through gifts of money. Karen was deeply hurt by what she experienced as a series of rebuffs when she attempted to reach out to him on a more intimate level. Yet when I tried to help her strategize ways to communicate with him about her desire for them to have a closer, more affectionate relationship, she would quickly shut down emotionally.

At the end of one session, the following exchange took place. [*Note: the ellipses indicate the pace at which therapist and client sent their text messages.*]

Karen: It doesn't seem like you can get close to my dad . . . his help now is monetary, like it's the only way he knows how to reach out to me.

Therapist: And how do you feel about that?

Karen: Let down, that it's all we have for a relationship . . . but I know that is all we have, it's all we have ever had, it seems. . . . I would give anything to have a relationship with him instead of his money.

Therapist: Have you ever been able to say that to him?

Karen: No, I don't think I ever could.

Therapist: We could consider it as a possible long-term goal.

Karen: I know it's time to stop. When do you want to meet next week?

Karen seemed in a hurry to end the session at this point. The online therapist develops an intuitive sense of when the client is resisting, which may be expressed in text, in emoticons, or in silence and the timing of communication. The following week, Karen both acknowledged her resistance and described her ongoing process.

Karen: I thought about telling my father I want [a relationship to him and not his money] . . . I can't imagine wanting or needing to say that to him . . . it would be so hurtful . . . . it's like he is oblivious to his ways and our relationship . . . it seems like we are unable to connect emotionally . . . it just seems like a waste of energy trying to get close to someone that seems emotionally unavailable.

At this point, I suggested that Karen try to make a distinction between what was practical or possible and what she really felt and longed for.

Therapist: It sounds like you're having difficulty reaching for a sense of what you really want . . . because your practical, reasoning side says . . . this man can't change (any more than he already has by not drinking) . . . so I might as well not get in touch with how I wish my father was.

Karen: I feel like I am grieving for my dad . . . or for my relationship (or lack of) with him.

We then explored what kind of response she wished her father could give. The client experienced immediate feelings and shared them with the therapist.

Karen: I have reached and reached and reached for him . . . and he has never grabbed for me.

Therapist: How do you picture that moment–if he could respond?

Karen: It makes me cry just thinking about it . . . it would be so great to really feel like I had his love.

Like their counterparts in face-to-face practice, online therapists and clients can form an intense and productive therapeutic relationship, share corrective experiences, process feelings, and achieve emotional growth. Addictions therapists with the skills to identify and work with partners and adult children of alcoholics are uniquely prepared to help the many isolated and fearful individuals who won't walk into a therapist's office or a 12-step meeting, but will risk a cry for help in text from the safety of their home.

Index

BOOK ORDER FORM!

Order a copy of this book with this form or online at:
http://www.HaworthPress.com/store/product.asp?sku= 5871

Impact of Substance Abuse on Children and Families
Research and Practice Implications

___ in softbound at $19.95 ISBN-13: 978-0-7890-3344-4 / ISBN-10: 0-7890-3344-5.
___ in hardbound at $39.95 ISBN-13: 978-0-7890-3343-7 / ISBN-10: 0-7890-3343-7.

COST OF BOOKS _____

POSTAGE & HANDLING _____
US: $4.00 for first book & $1.50
   for each additional book
Outside US: $5.00 for first book
& $2.00 for each additional book.

SUBTOTAL _____

In Canada: add 7% GST._____

STATE TAX _____
CA, IL, IN, MN, NJ, NY, OH, PA & SD residents
please add appropriate local sales tax.

FINAL TOTAL _____

If paying in Canadian funds, convert
using the current exchange rate,
UNESCO coupons welcome.

❑ BILL ME LATER:
Bill-me option is good on US/Canada/
Mexico orders only; not good to jobbers,
wholesalers, or subscription agencies.

❑ Signature _____

❑ Payment Enclosed: $_____

❑ PLEASE CHARGE TO MY CREDIT CARD:

❑ Visa ❑ MasterCard ❑ AmEx ❑ Discover
❑ Diner's Club ❑ Eurocard ❑ JCB

Account #_____

Exp Date_____

Signature_____
(Prices in US dollars and subject to change without notice.)

PLEASE PRINT ALL INFORMATION OR ATTACH YOUR BUSINESS CARD

Name _____

Address _____

City _____ State/Province _____ Zip/Postal Code _____

Country _____

Tel _____ Fax _____

E-Mail _____

May we use your e-mail address for confirmations and other types of information? ❑ Yes ❑ No We appreciate receiving
your e-mail address. Haworth would like to e-mail special discount offers to you, as a preferred customer.
We will never share, rent, or exchange your e-mail address. We regard such actions as an invasion of your privacy.

Order from your **local bookstore** or directly from
The Haworth Press, Inc. 10 Alice Street, Binghamton, New York 13904-1580 • USA
Call our toll-free number (1-800-429-6784) / Outside US/Canada: (607) 722-5857
Fax: 1-800-895-0582 / Outside US/Canada: (607) 771-0012
E-mail your order to us: orders@HaworthPress.com
For orders outside US and Canada, you may wish to order through your local
sales representative, distributor, or bookseller.
For information, see http://HaworthPress.com/distributors

(Discounts are available for individual orders in US and Canada only, not booksellers/distributors.)

Please photocopy this form for your personal use.
www.HaworthPress.com

BOF06